LEM

MAR 1 8 1996	DATE DUE	
NOV 08 1996	NOV 22 1999	JAN 1 8 '08
NOV 22 1996	DEC 10 1999	APR 2 2 '09
DEC 1 2 1996	JA 06 '00	MAR 0 2 '10
JAN 02 1996	AP 12 '00	OCT 1 2 '10
FEB 07 1997	MR 06 '01	NOV 1 8 '11
MAR 10 1997	TO 06 '01	DEC 1 6 '11
ILL 96/97	MR 04 '02	
MAY 12 1997	FE 16 '04	
ILL. 97/98	NA	
MAY 1 5 1998	JA 31 '05	
FEB 0 4 1999	OC 04 '07	

MARIO LEMIEUX

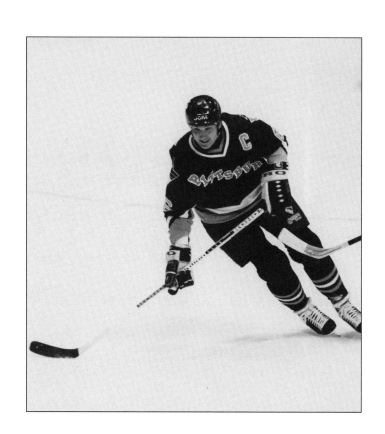

GREAT ACHIEVERS:
LIVES OF THE PHYSICALLY CHALLENGED

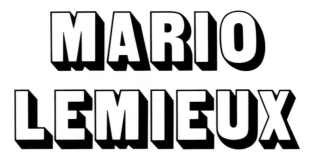

ICE HOCKEY STAR

Jeff Z. Klein

Chelsea House Publishers

New York • Philadelphia

CHELSEA HOUSE PUBLISHERS

EDITORIAL DIRECTOR   Richard Rennert
EXECUTIVE MANAGING EDITOR   Karyn Gullen Browne
COPY CHIEF   Robin James
PICTURE EDITOR   Adrian G. Allen
CREATIVE DIRECTOR   Robert Mitchell
ART DIRECTOR   Joan Ferrigno
MANUFACTURING DIRECTOR   Gerald Levine

GREAT ACHIEVERS: LIVES OF THE PHYSICALLY CHALLENGED

SENIOR EDITOR   Kathy Kuhtz Campbell
SERIES DESIGN   Basia Niemczyc

Staff for **MARIO LEMIEUX**
ASSISTANT EDITOR   Joy Sanchez
EDITORIAL ASSISTANT   Scott D. Briggs
PICTURE RESEARCHER   Matthew Dudley
COVER ILLUSTRATION   Jon Weiman

First Printing

1   3   5   7   9   8   6   4   2

Library of Congress Cataloging-in-Publication Data

Klein, Jeff Z.
Mario Lemieux, ice hockey star / Jeff Z. Klein.
p. cm.—(Great achievers)
Includes bibliographical references and index.
ISBN 0-7910-7910-2400-8
        0-7910-2401-6 (pbk.)
1. Lemieux, Mario, 1965– —Juvenile literature. 2. Hockey players— Canada—
Biography—Juvenile literature. 3. Hodgkin's disease—Patients— Canada—
Biography—Juvenile literature. 4. Pittsburgh Penguins (Hockey team)—Juvenile
literature.

[1. Lemieux, Mario, 1965–. 2. Hockey players. 3. Hodgkin's disease. 4. Diseases.] I.
Title. II. Series: Great achievers (Chelsea House Publishers)
GV848.5.L46K54 1995   94-31522
796.962'092—dc20   CIP
[B]   AC

FRONTISPIECE

Pittsburgh Penguins center Mario Lemieux, looking in fine form on March 2, 1993, at the first game he played after undergoing radiation treatments for Hodgkin's disease.

CONTENTS

GREAT ACHIEVERS

LIVES OF THE PHYSICALLY CHALLENGED

A MESSAGE FOR EVERYONE

Jerry Lewis

Just 44 years ago—when I was the ripe old age of 23—an incredible stroke of fate rocketed me to overnight stardom as an entertainer. After the initial shock wore off, I began to have a very strong feeling that, in return for all life had given me, I must find a way of giving something back. At just that moment, a deeply moving experience in my personal life persuaded me to take up the leadership of a fledgling battle to defeat a then little-known group of diseases called muscular dystrophy, as well as other related neuromuscular diseases—all of which are disabling and, in the worst cases, cut life short.

In 1950, when the Muscular Dystrophy Association (MDA)—of which I am national chairman—was established, physical disability was looked on as a matter of shame. Franklin Roosevelt, who guided America through World War II from a wheelchair, and Harold Russell, the World War II hero who lost both hands in battle, then became an Academy Award–winning movie star and chairman of the President's Committee on Employment of the Handicapped, were the exceptions. One of the reasons that muscular dystrophy and related diseases were so little known was that people who had been disabled by them were hidden at home, away from the pity and discomfort with which they were generally regarded by society. As I got to know and began working with people who have disabilities, I quickly learned what a tragic mistake this perception was. And my determination to correct this terrible problem soon became as great as my commitment to see disabling neuromuscular diseases wiped from the face of the earth.

I have long wondered why it never occurs to us, as we experience the knee-jerk inclination to feel sorry for people who are physically disabled, that lives such as those led by President Roosevelt, Harold Russell, and all of the extraordinary people profiled in this Great Achievers series demonstrate unmistakably how wrong we are. Physical disability need not be something that blights life and destroys opportunity for personal fulfillment and accomplishment. On the contrary, as people such as Ray Charles, Stephen Hawking, and Ron Kovic prove, physical disability can be a spur to greatness rather than a condemnation of emptiness.

In fact, if my experience with physically disabled people can be taken as a guide, as far as accomplishment is concerned, they have a slight edge on the rest of us. The unusual challenges they face require finding greater-than-average sources of energy and determination to achieve much of what able-bodied people take for granted. Often, this ultimately translates into a lifetime of superior performance in whatever endeavor people with disabilities choose to pursue.

If you have watched my Labor Day Telethon over the years, you know exactly what I am talking about. Annually, we introduce to tens of millions of Americans people whose accomplishments would distinguish them regardless of their physical conditions—top-ranking executives, physicians, scientists, lawyers, musicians, and artists. The message I hope the audience receives is not that these extraordinary individuals have achieved what they have by overcoming a dreadful disadvantage that the rest of us are lucky not to have to endure. Rather, I hope our viewers reflect on the fact that these outstanding people have been ennobled and strengthened by the tremendous challenges they have faced.

In 1992, MDA, which has grown over the past four decades into one of the world's leading voluntary health agencies, established a personal achievement awards program to demonstrate to the nation that the distinctive qualities of people with disabilities are by no means confined to the famous. What could have been more appropriate or timely in that year of the implementation of the 1990 Americans with Disabilities Act than to take an action that could perhaps finally achieve the alteration of public perception of disability, which MDA had struggled over four decades to achieve?

On Labor Day, 1992, it was my privilege to introduce to America MDA's inaugural national personal achievement award winner, Steve Mikita, assistant attorney general of the state of Utah. Steve graduated magna cum laude from Duke University as its first wheelchair student in history and was subsequently named the outstanding young lawyer of the year by the Utah Bar Association. After he spoke on the Telethon with an eloquence that caused phones to light up from coast to coast, people asked me where he had been all this time and why they had not known of him before, so deeply impressed were they by him. I answered that he and thousands like him have been here all along. We just have not adequately *noticed* them.

It is my fervent hope that we can eliminate indifference once and for all and make it possible for all of our fellow citizens with disabilities to gain their rightfully high place in our society.

ON FACING CHALLENGES

John Callahan

I was paralyzed for life in 1972, at the age of 21. A friend and I were driving in a Volkswagen on a hot July night, when he smashed the car at full speed into a utility pole. He suffered only minor injuries. But my spinal cord was severed during the crash, leaving me without any feeling from my diaphragm downward. The only muscles I could move were some in my upper body and arms, and I could also extend my fingers. After spending a lot of time in physical therapy, it became possible for me to grasp a pen.

I've always loved to draw. When I was a kid, I made pictures of everything from Daffy Duck (one of my lifelong role models) to caricatures of my teachers and friends. I've always been a people watcher, it seems; and I've always looked at the world in a sort of skewed way. Everything I see just happens to translate immediately into humor. And so, humor has become my way of coping. As the years have gone by, I have developed a tremendous drive to express my humor by drawing cartoons.

The key to cartooning is to put a different spin on the expected, the normal. And that's one reason why many of my cartoons deal with the disabled: amputees, quadriplegics, paraplegics, the blind. The public is not used to seeing them in cartoons.

But there's another reason why my subjects are often disabled men and women. I'm sick and tired of people who presume to speak for the disabled. Call me a cripple, call me a gimp, call me paralyzed for life.

Just don't call me something I'm not. I'm not "differently abled," and my cartoons show that disabled people should not be treated any differently than anyone else.

All of the men, women, and children who are profiled in the Great Achievers series share this in common: their various handicaps have not prevented them from accomplishing great things. Their life stories are worth knowing about because they have found the strength and courage to develop their talents and to follow their dreams as fully as they can.

Whether able-bodied or disabled, a person must strive to overcome obstacles. There's nothing greater than to see a person who faces challenges and conquers them, regardless of his or her limitations.

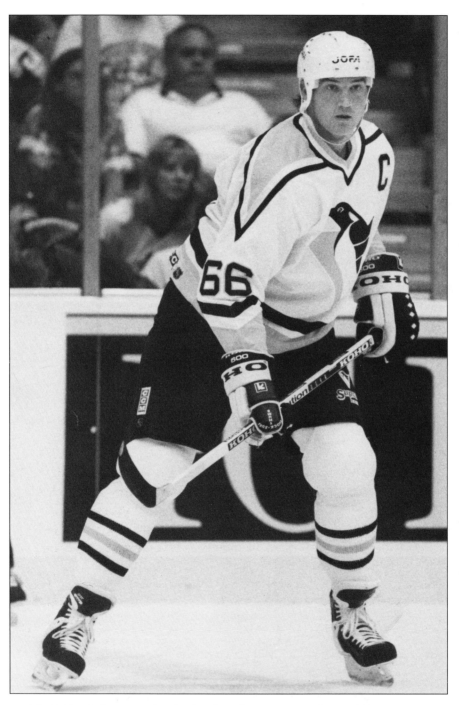

Mario Lemieux, center for the Pittsburgh Penguins and one of the greatest hockey players of all time, was diagnosed with Hodgkin's disease, or cancer of the lymphatic system, in January 1993.

1

"THE TOUGHEST DAY OF MY LIFE"

THE NEWS SPREAD like wildfire ever since it had been first announced on January 12, 1993. Mario Lemieux—the 27-year-old superstar center of the Pittsburgh Penguins and three-time scoring champion of the National Hockey League (NHL); the man who led the Penguins to the Stanley Cup the last two years and was now en route to shattering hockey great Wayne Gretzky's seemingly unbreakable single-season scoring records—had cancer.

On January 15, 150 reporters streamed into a hotel ballroom in downtown Pittsburgh, Pennsylvania, to hear Lemieux's first public statement about his condition. More than a dozen television cameramen and two dozen still photographers stood ready to capture the news conference proceedings, which would be carried live on all three of Pittsburgh's commercial TV stations, a French-language station in Lemieux's hometown of Montreal, Quebec, and a Canadian English-language sports network.

The principals strode to the dais: Penguins team president Howard Baldwin, general manager Craig Patrick, and coach Scotty Bowman; NHL president Gil Stein; Lemieux's two physicians, Charles Burke and Theodore Crandall; and finally, Lemieux himself. The room fell silent except for the clicking and whirring of the cameras. Lemieux spoke.

> Any time you hear the word cancer, it's a scary thing. When the doctors gave me the news, I could hardly drive home because of the tears, and I was crying the whole day. That certainly was the toughest day of my life.

Mario Lemieux speaks at a press conference on January 15, 1993, in Pittsburgh, Pennsylvania, giving his first public statement about having Hodgkin's disease.

Lemieux went on to describe how a year and a half before he had first noticed a tiny lump in his neck. He had thought nothing of it for a long time, but recently he

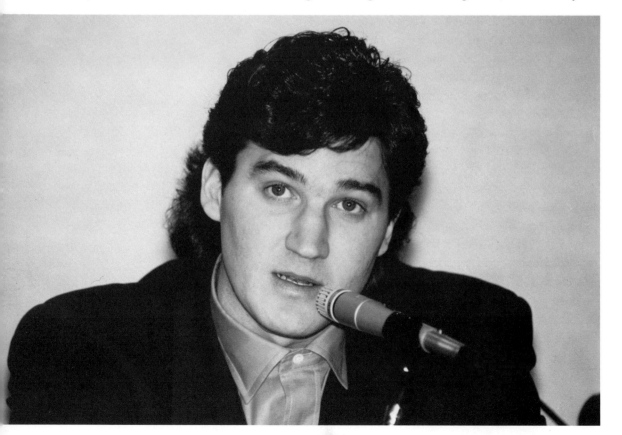

had realized that it had grown. Finally, in December 1992, he told Burke, the Penguins team doctor, about it. Dr. Burke did not think it was anything to worry about, but recommended that Lemieux have it examined if he wanted. Lemieux did. The one-by-two-centimeter lump was removed from his neck on Friday, January 8, 1993. On Saturday, the results were in. The lump was cancerous. Mario Lemieux had Hodgkin's disease — cancer of the lymph nodes.

Crandall, the oncologist (cancer specialist) in charge of Lemieux's treatment, and Burke told the reporters that because the lump was found in the initial stage of its development, the outlook was good. Hodgkin's disease, they said, was curable in 90 to 95 percent of cases when found early.

Lemieux answered questions from reporters in English, his adopted language, and in French, his mother tongue. How did his teammates react? "I walked in the room," answered Lemieux, "and everybody was silent. That's not like our team. It was tough for everybody. I wasn't sure what to say, and nobody else knew what to say. I've had the same experience, talking to people with cancer and not knowing what to say, except, Good luck."

Was the June wedding to his longtime girlfriend, Nathalie Asselin, who was pregnant with their first child, still on? "Yes," said Lemieux.

Would he be back in time for the Stanley Cup playoffs in April? Perhaps, said Lemieux, but "the time frame is not important to any of us here. I'll be back when I'm 100 percent cured. In six weeks, eight weeks, next year. That's not important."

Lemieux, a very private man known for not saying much to reporters during his nine years of international hockey superstardom, spoke at length, even smiling on occasion, as he outlined how he would approach this crisis. "I'm a positive person by nature," he said, "and that's not going to change in the future even though I have Hodgkin's.

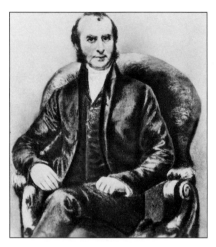

Hodgkin's disease was named after Thomas Hodgkin, the British doctor who first detected cancer of the lymphatic system in 1832. It is a relatively rare form of cancer that most commonly affects males between the ages of 20 and 40.

That's not going to change my life and the way I live my life. Certainly it's going to make it tougher for the next couple of months, but that's life sometimes. Sometimes in life, you have to go through tough periods. . . . But you climb the mountain. We know this disease is curable."

Lemieux was asked to talk about the other people he knew who had been diagnosed with cancer. Two of his uncles, he replied, had died of cancer, and a cousin had died of Hodgkin's disease. The sister-in-law of his agent, Tom Reich, had also passed away due to cancer. And, of course, Bob Johnson, the former coach of the Penguins, had died of brain cancer a few months after they had won their first Stanley Cup in 1991. Then, too, there were all the patients Lemieux had visited as honorary chairman of the Pittsburgh Cancer Institute for the previous five years. "I'm not the type who enjoys doing it," said Lemieux, who admitted that he no longer went very often. "You have to toughen yourself to visit a patient. Now, a couple years later, I'm faced with the same thing."

Crandall told reporters that Lemieux faced a month of five-days-a-week radiation treatments, but that they could not begin for two weeks because Lemieux currently had a minor lung infection unrelated to the Hodgkin's. Once the radiation therapy began, Crandall continued, Lemieux could possibly experience fatigue and other side effects and might not be ready to play again for several weeks after the treatments concluded. And as is the case with most forms of cancer, no one is considered fully cured until five years have elapsed without a recurrence of the disease. Still, Crandall emphasized, the outlook for Lemieux was quite good.

Hodgkin's disease, it would later be noted in articles written about Lemieux's condition, is a cancer that most frequently affects young males. It attacks the lymphatic system, which protects the body from infection. The swollen neck glands people often experience while suffering from colds or other common illnesses are an indication that the system is at work warding off infection. The lymphatic system consists of the network of vessels that suffuse body tissue, as well as the bone marrow, tonsils, thymus, spleen, and the tiny organs known as lymph nodes. In Lemieux's case, a swollen lymph node was what led to discovering the cancer.

Although what causes it remains a mystery, the disease—named for Thomas Hodgkin, the British doctor who first detected it in 1832—is relatively rare. Only 1 percent of all cancers in the United States are classified as Hodgkin's, which translates to roughly 8,000 cases per year. However the cancer is treated—whether through radiation therapy, the use of anticancer drugs, or a combination of both—it is imperative that the cancer be stopped before it spreads to and destroys other organs in the patient's body.

The press conference concluded and the people adjourned. Lemieux made his way through the crowd. When he reached the exit, he paused to shake hands with several fans who had gathered to show their support for Pittsburgh's most popular athlete. He smiled and thanked them for their concern. Meanwhile, a reporter asked Crandall whether, since the early-stage cure rate for Hodgkin's is so high, maybe too big a deal was being made of all this.

"Cancer," replied Crandall, "is cancer."

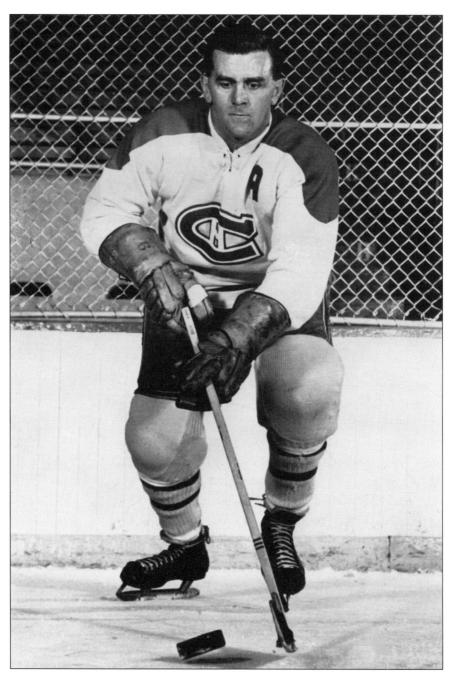

Maurice "Rocket" Richard, the star player for the Montreal Canadiens in the 1940s and 1950s, was suspended in 1955 for fighting, which incited mobs of fans to set fires and smash store windows outside the Montreal Forum. The uproar became known as the Richard Riot.

2

THE CATHEDRAL
OF HOCKEY

MARIO LEMIEUX was born on October 5, 1965, in the working-class Montreal neighborhood of Ville Emard. His father, the stoic Jean-Guy, was a house builder and fervent fan of the Montreal Canadiens hockey team. His mother, the outgoing Pierrette, was also a big fan of *le club de hockey Canadien.* Mario had two brothers. Alain was five years older than Mario, and Richard was one and a half years older. Like them, he was holding a hockey stick before he could walk, and by the time he was three, he was playing the game on skates.

The idea of a Canadian boy playing ice hockey at age three is not at all unusual. Ever since hockey rules were codified in the late 19th century, it has been the nation's most popular sport and one of its most culturally distinctive icons. Nothing is more Canadian than a hockey game, even though the sport has long since spread and developed a slightly different flavor in the United States, Europe, and beyond.

But no matter where hockey is played, Montreal is revered as its mecca, and not just because the first organized league was formed there in 1875. Three of the greatest early-era teams were based in Montreal—the Montreal Amateur Athletic Association, winners of the Stanley Cup in 1893, 1894, and 1902; the Montreal Victorias, Stanley Cup winners in 1895, 1897, 1898, and 1899; and the Montreal Wanderers, Cup winners in 1906, 1907, 1908, and 1910. And a very high percentage of the professional and top amateur players of that era came from Montreal, Canada's largest city since the middle of the 19th century.

The Stanley Cup is the trophy awarded annually to the winning team of the National Hockey League playoffs. It was first presented to the Canadian amateur champions in 1893 by Lord Stanley of Preston, the governor-general of Canada. With the rise of professionalism in the first years of the 20th Century, the champions of the various pro

The first hockey league was formed in Montreal, Canada, in 1875. Two of the greatest hockey teams of this time were based in Montreal—the Amateur Athletic Association and the Wanderers. This picture depicts an 1895 hockey match at the city's Victoria Rink.

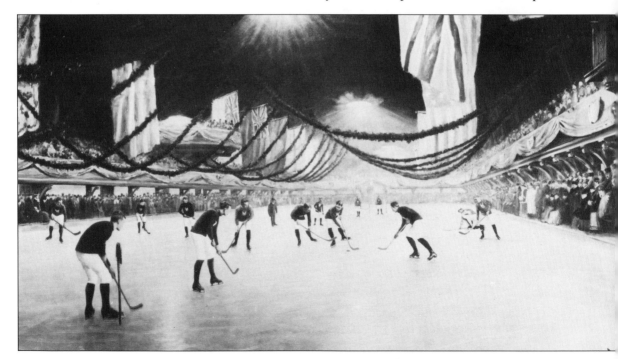

leagues vied for the Cup. Finally, in 1926, only one major pro league remained—the NHL. Ever since that 1926–27 season, the Cup has been presented to the champions of the NHL.

Ultimately, what cemented Montreal's place at the center of the hockey universe was the Canadiens. In 1909 the club was founded with the specific purpose of representing the city's French-speaking majority. With the Wanderers and the Victorias more or less representing Montreal's English-speaking elite, and the less successful Shamrocks (who won the Stanley Cup in 1900 only) being the club of the city's sizable Irish population, the Canadiens filled a very important—and large—niche in the passionate world of Montreal hockey.

The Canadiens became so popular that they helped drive the other two teams out of existence. (Eventually the Canadiens came to be known as the Habs—short for *habitants,* the French word for "inhabitant" and what the Quebecois have called themselves since the 1500s.) They were the Stanley Cup champions in 1916, and by 1917, the first year of play after the formation of the NHL, they were the only team representing Montreal at the highest level of professional hockey. In 1924 they won their second Stanley Cup.

Throughout this period the Canadiens' management carefully cultivated the club's image. In the beginning, playing to a predominantly French-speaking audience, the Habs' first big stars were the classy captain Jack Laviolette, the deft *wingman* Didier Pitre, the cool goalie Georges Vezina, and the high scoring but vicious Edouard "Newsy" Lalonde. Later, as the club became the standard-bearer for all of Montreal, an effort was made to appeal to and reflect the city as a whole. Thus, it was important to have French-speaking stars, but now English-speaking players were more than welcome. By the mid-1920s, the best and most popular Habs were English-speaking Howie

Morenz, from Stratford, Ontario, and the bilingual Aurel Joliat, from Ottawa, Ontario.

In 1924 a group of Canadian businessmen tried to recapture the English-speaking segment of Montreal's hockey fandom. They founded the Montreal Maroons, and stocked the club almost exclusively with English-speaking players. The Maroons were a good team, capturing the Stanley Cup at the end of the 1925–26 season, the second year of their existence. That year also happened to be the opening season for the big new building that both teams shared: the Montreal Forum.

Standing in the heart of downtown on the rue Ste. Catherine, the Forum, with a capacity of more than 12,000, was one of the largest auditoriums in North America. It would not be long before the hockey world would revere the Forum as its shrine in much the same way that New York's Yankee Stadium or London's Wembley Stadium would be regarded as the shrines of baseball and soccer.

Over the next dozen years the Canadiens and Maroons enjoyed a spirited rivalry based on the ethnic differences of the city, with the Habs winning two Stanley Cups and four divisional titles, and the Maroons taking one Stanley Cup, in 1935, and two divisional crowns. But in 1938, during the lean years of the Great Depression, the Maroons folded. Le Canadien, as the Quebecois still call the Canadiens, have reigned over Montreal unchallenged ever since.

But it was not until the 1940s that the Forum and the Habs began to take on the near-mystical aura they have today. In 1942, a young Quebecois joined the Canadiens, a 21-year-old with slicked-back jet black hair and eyes that were always compared to burning coals. His name was Maurice Richard, and he had a hot temper and a burning hunger for goal, which he expressed in lightning rushes around, through, and over opposing players. His outbursts of anger were sometimes remarkably violent, even in a game that featured frequent fistfights and bloodcurdling stick fouls.

In 1944–45, Richard scored 50 goals during the 50-game schedule. True, the league as a whole had been weakened because many players were serving as soldiers, sailors, and airmen in World War II, but no one had scored a goal per game since Bill Cook and Dick Irvin potted 32 and 30, respectively, in the 30-game Western League season of 1925–26. "Rocket" Richard's feat electrified the hockey world.

By 1954, the Habs had won four regular-season titles and three Stanley Cup championships during the Richard years. As the end of the 1954–55 season approached, the Habs seemed headed for another regular-season crown and perhaps another Cup. But in the fourth game from the end of the season, Richard went berserk, getting into a fight with two Chicago Black Hawks, slashing one with a stick, then striking a *linesman* who tried to break it up. NHL

Montreal, today a city of 2.4 million people in southern Quebec, Canada, is considered to be the hub of ice hockey. The city is the home of the Canadiens and the birthplace of Mario Lemieux.

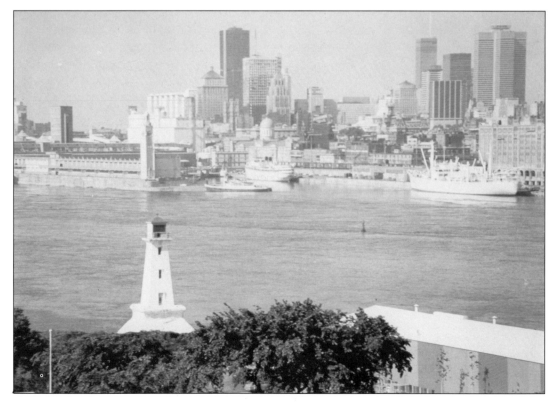

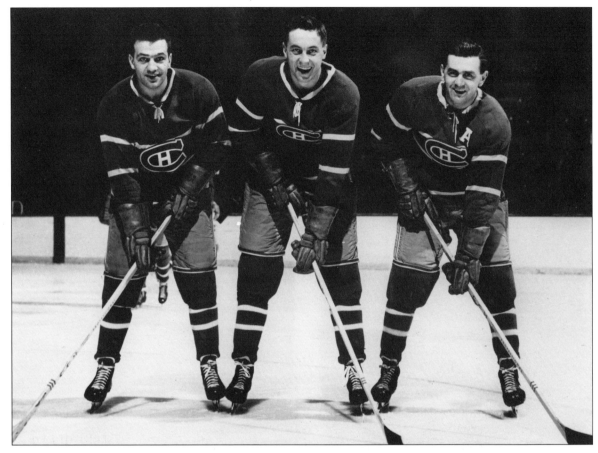

Montreal Canadiens legends (left to right) Bernie "Boom Boom" Geoffrion, Jean Béliveau, and Rocket Richard pose with their sticks on March 4, 1955. The following season the Canadiens won the first of five straight Stanley Cups.

president Clarence Campbell reacted by suspending the Rocket for the rest of the season and the playoffs.

Montreal fans thought the suspension was much too stiff. They were outraged that Campbell was depriving the Habs of their best, most charismatic player for the duration of the hockey year. There was also an unmistakable ethnic component to all this. Many French-speaking Montrealers regarded Campbell as an example of English Canadian authority seeking to keep a French Canadian icon in his place—volatile symbolism at a time when francophone (French-speaking) Quebecers were increasingly coming to believe that they were second-class citizens in their own province.

The crowd was already in a restive mood when Campbell took his usual seat at the Forum for the regular-season finale. They shouted insults at him and showered him with debris. A fan came up and punched him, and someone threw a smoke bomb. The building was evacuated and the game forfeited.

Outside the Forum, a mob formed and ran up and down rue Ste. Catherine, smashing store windows, setting fires, and overturning cars. Dozens were arrested, but order was not fully restored until Richard himself went on the radio later that night and appealed for calm. The disturbance became known as the Richard Riot, and many Canadian observers believe it was a key event in the development of Quebec nationalism.

One oft-cited reason for the rise in Quebecois cultural awareness was the urbanization of the province, as thousands began to move from farms into the cities. Jean-Guy Lemieux, at age 18, was part of that population shift, moving from a farm in rural Quebec to Montreal in the early 1950s. Already ensconced in the two-storied house on rue Jorgue, he and Pierrette moved into the downstairs flat while his mother lived upstairs.

The Lemieuxs did not have a lot of money, but most Saturday nights Jean-Guy and sometimes Pierrette made the 10-minute walk to the Forum to buy a ticket to see Le Canadien. Jean-Guy even bought season tickets for the 1955–56 season.

He could not have chosen a better time. That year the Canadiens won the first of five straight Stanley Cups—a feat that to this day has never been matched. Now the Habs were being hailed as the Flying Frenchmen by the English and Les Glorieux by the French. Admired by all for their speed and panache, they still had Rocket Richard, but he was joined by his little brother Henri ("The Pocket Rocket"), Bernie "Boom Boom" Geoffrion, and the future on-ice leader of the team, Jean Béliveau. To be French Canadian in the 1950s and 1960s, one almost had to love

Le Canadien. The fans' embrace of the team, coming at a time when the Quebecois were embracing a new sense of their own culture, was complete and virtually religious. As Clark Blaise wrote in his short story, "I'm Dreaming of Rocket Richard":

> The ice of big-time hockey, the old Forum . . . Something about the ghostly white of the ice under those powerful lights, something about the hiss of the skates if you were standing close enough, the solid pock-pock of the rubber on the sticks, and the low menacing whiz of a Rocket wrist-shot hugging the ice—there was nothing in any other sport to compare to the spell of hockey. Inside the Forum in the early '50s, those games . . . were evangelical, for truly we were dans le cénacle [in the chamber], where everyone breathed as one.

Thus, in the year of Mario Lemieux's birth, for Montreal—a city of 2.4 million, two-thirds of whom were French Canadian—hockey was more than merely an obsession; it was almost a cultural duty. It was a game played by everyone: on makeshift ice rinks in vacant lots during the long winters, on the streets, and in indoor rinks year-round. But the Lemieux household on rue Jorgue came up with the most remarkable ice rink of all.

One winter when her three boys were still little, Pierrette wondered where they could play; she did not want them walking the two blocks to the nearby outdoor rink at St. Jean de Matha Church, and she did not want them running around in the busy street. Then she hit upon the idea of using the family living room. Enlisting Jean-Guy's help, they hauled in enough snow to cover the entire living room rug, packed it down hard, and opened all the windows and doors. Soon, they had a miniature indoor rink that, while several steps below the Forum in terms of ice quality, served the family's purposes quite nicely.

Pierrette and Jean-Guy helped the boys into their skates, and soon the five of them were sloshing through the living room snow. "They were so young they were skating more

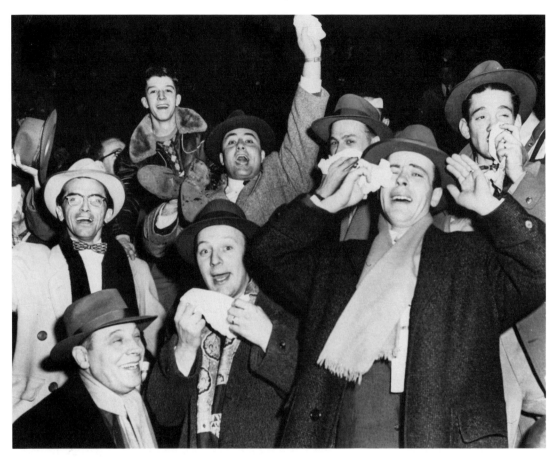

on the boots than on the blades," Pierrette later told author Jean Sonmor. "But it was fun; I would have played too if I could have. All I could do was play goal." It was a scene repeated perhaps a half-dozen times in Mario's early childhood.

Mario was skating with a puck and stick by age three, and a year later he was playing with his brothers all afternoon and into the night at St. Jean de Matha, whose rink, like countless church rinks throughout the predominantly Catholic province, hosted both organized and pickup games all winter long. He was already developing the skills that would, from an early age, set him apart from every other hockey player on the face of the earth.

Canadiens fans have always been passionate about their team. The emotional crowd at the Montreal Forum cries and yells during the first period of a game between the Canadiens and the Detroit Red Wings on March 18, 1955.

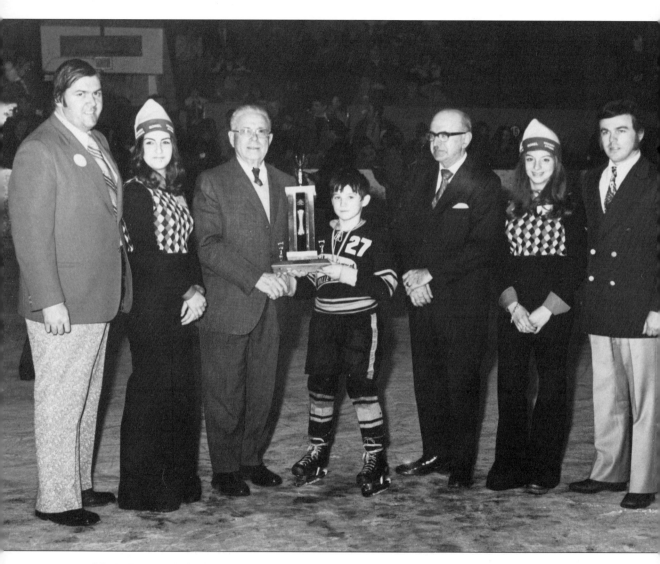

Mario Lemieux's hockey prowess was evident at a young age. He is seen here as a six-year-old, after he won the Most Valuable Player Award at a provincial tournament in Sorel, Quebec, where he scored 11 goals and 11 assists.

3

THE PRODIGY

THE FIRST SIGN of Mario Lemieux's hockey greatness was spotted when he was just four years old. Under the watchful eye of a local hockey instructor named Fernand Fichaud, Mario was involved in a skate-around with a few other boys his age—the type of activity that usually results in all the children falling down and struggling to get back up again. But Fichaud watched in amazement as Mario skated with the puck, moved past a couple of boys, then headed for the net. Shifting his weight from side to side, Mario had the goalie dropping to one end of the net, when suddenly he pulled from right to left, then deposited the puck into the now-vacant net. He had *deked* the goalie right out of the play.

Fichaud knew this was something an older boy might be able to do, but not a four-year-old. Fichaud later told author Lawrence Martin: "I think about that move all my life. That was the greatest thing I ever saw. His parents knew how extraordinary it was. They could tell what it meant."

At age six, Mario was a *center* on an "atom" team, as the squads for that age group are called in Canadian youth hockey terminology. In a Quebec provincial tournament, he dominated play and was voted most valuable player and most likely to succeed. Soon the word was out about the child prodigy from Ville Emard. An atom game featuring Mario drew some 5,000 spectators. A championship game drew 5,000. He scored goals by the bushel, thanks to his uncanny stickhandling ability and the hard shot of a boy twice his age.

In adulthood, Lemieux would be known for these qualities and for his size. As an adult measuring six feet four inches and weighing 210 pounds, Lemieux would be one of the NHL's biggest players. But as a youth, he was average sized and ordinary—until he got the puck on the end of his stick.

Mario's brothers were good players, too. The oldest, Alain, was a swift and talented *forward* who would eventually make it all the way to the NHL for a brief but respectable career. Richard was big and not much of a skater, but in his youth hockey days he was a good *defenseman* whose heavy shot was said to be very impressive.

Mario, as a young phenom wearing number 27 (the same number Alain wore) for the Ville Emard Hurricanes, moved up through the age group divisions. He won individual scoring titles while leading Ville Emard to team championships each year. All along, he showed an uncanny sense of what was happening on the ice around him. The story is told about how one day in practice Mario laid a perfect *drop pass* onto the stick of a trailing teammate, even though the teammate had never called for the puck and Mario had never once looked behind him. How, asked the coach, did you know he was there? "I could tell by the sound of his skates," replied Mario.

The peewee level begins at age 11, and it is at this stage in youth hockey that hitting is first allowed. Here, some people thought, Mario would get his first real test. Could he stand up to the *bodychecking* that he would inevitably attract as the team's biggest offensive weapon?

His first peewee game was against Notre Dame de Grace, a hard-hitting team that attacked Mario all night.

Through the years, Mario led the Ville Emard Hurricanes to victory each season. Nine-year-old Mario (far right) and his teammates pose for the camera after winning the 1974 Tom Thumb hockey tournament.

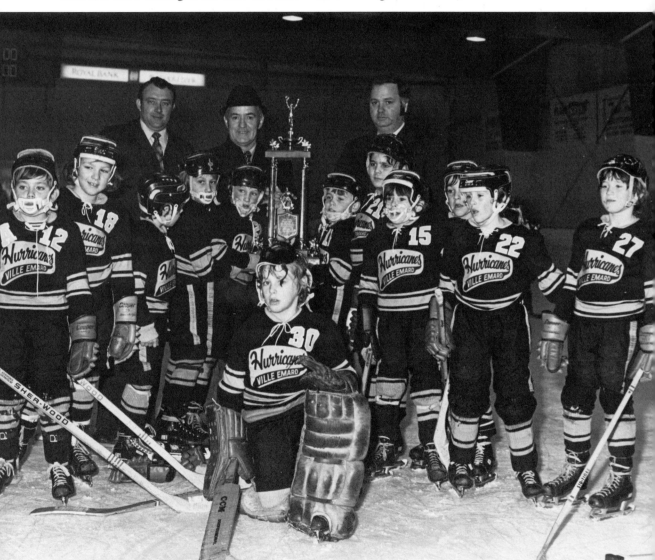

But they could not stop him. Mario scored eight goals that night, leading Ville Emard to victory. Subsequently, he would draw a lot of bodychecking attention, and some illegal stickwork as well. In addition, some parents in the stands harassed Mario. On more than one occasion, the parents of opposing players spit at him.

In response to all this, Mario developed some gamesmanship tactics of his own. He would chop at opponents with his stick, doling out two-handed slashes at the players checking him. In one tournament for the provincial peewee championship, Mario took so many retaliatory *penalties* that his coaches benched him. Frustrated, he broke down and cried in the dressing room during the second intermission. He was finally put back into the game and helped Ville Emard rally for a win. In another game, he was benched again for retaliating too often. Ville Emard fell behind 6–1. He was put back on the ice for the third *period* and scored six goals in the final session to lead the Hurricanes to a 7–6 victory.

Mario took hockey seriously. He needed to win in order to be happy. His father, watching Mario from the stands playing against one team or another, would only be content if Mario scored three or four goals in one game. At that time alone would a smile cross Jean-Guy's face. Mario's determination and competitive edge would carry over to other parts of his life, especially when playing a game of cards or Monopoly at home. His father commented, "If Mario lost, it would be like a hurricane went through the basement."

All along, Mario had the full and nurturing support of his family. People who knew the Lemieuxs were impressed with how close-knit they were and noticed how indulgent the parents were—particularly Pierrette—with the boys. They were spoiled by their mother and were used to getting their way. According to one family legend, when Mario was eight years old, he, Richard, and Alain wanted to watch "Soirée de Hockey," the televised Saturday night hockey game that is a staple of Canadian life. When the baby-sitter would not change the channel from the program she was watching, the boys simply locked her in the bathroom until the game was over.

People wondered how Jean-Guy and Pierrette could have produced such fine athletes when they themselves had never been athletic. As a young man, Jean-Guy had suffered from lung ailments that limited his physical activity. But it is also true that Mario was never a particularly strong boy himself. Although never downright skinny like Wayne Gretzky was as a boy and a young man, Mario had relatively little upper-body strength, and was never particularly interested in building himself up. Like Gretzky, he simply possessed astonishing innate talent and extraordinary hockey sense. And he also seemed to know that for some hockey players, a sculpted muscular body is a pointless thing to have and can even be a hindrance, especially if it limits flexibility or somehow gets in the way of a deft touch. This seems contradictory in a game so rugged, but it is one of the mysteries of hockey that two of its greatest players, Gretzky and Lemieux, were never among the physically strongest players on their teams.

All hockey players, however, must have endurance. Mario's peewee coach, Ron Stevenson, made sure the Hurricanes had the leg and lung power they needed by putting them through tough practices. And however difficult those practices were, Mario never missed one of them in the four years he played for Stevenson.

At age 10, in his first year of peewee, Lemieux was one of three stars and future NHLers on the team with Jean-Jacques Daigneault and Marc Bergevin, both of whom were a year older. But in his second year, in which he would score a staggering 150 goals and 90 assists, Mario was named captain and shouldered new responsibilities. He did so quietly, for he said little on the way to the rink, in the dressing room, or during games. He never lost his temper with himself, his teammates, his opponents, or the referees in any outward, demonstrative way. Rather, his temper tended to smolder, and he would express his anger by scoring and setting up goals. "In four years I never had any trouble with him at all," Stevenson would later say of Mario. "My reward for 30 years of coaching hockey was the opportunity to coach Mario Lemieux. He was a great boy, as well as an outstanding player."

Mario's ability to restrain his temper took a great deal of forbearance, for he increasingly became the target of illegal stickwork and other overtly brutal tactics. But the Hurricanes had enforcers of their own, and they usually retaliated against the opposition just as hard in the roughly 100 games per season they played.

Already famous throughout Quebec, Mario had long since caught the notice of the Montreal Canadiens, who

Today, young Canadian boys still begin playing hockey at an early age. These children play hockey on the team that was once the Ville Emard Hurricanes, the club that Mario played for as a youth.

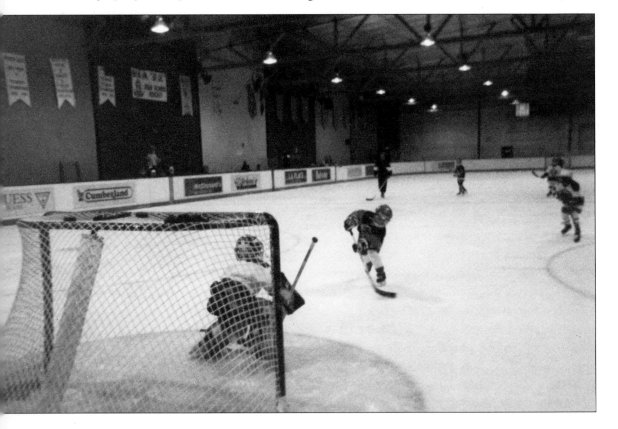

were in the midst of a four-year run as regular-season and Stanley Cup champions in the late 1970s. Coach Scotty Bowman called the 12-year-old Mario the greatest prospect he had ever seen. When Mario was honored as Montreal's youth player of the month, he got to sit behind the Habs' bench during a game. It turned out that it was the game in which Guy Lafleur—the latest in Les Glorieux's long line of Quebecois stars—scored his 500th goal. A photo in the next day's newspaper showed young Mario in the background as Lafleur is being congratulated by his teammates.

Once he reached the bantam level at age 14, Mario started to grow dramatically. By age 16, he had reached his full height and weighed 200 pounds. Now, he had size and mass to go along with his incredible skills. Mario seemed destined for superstardom, and Stevenson knew his young celebrity would have to deal with public demands that would be as challenging and insistent as anything he would face on the ice. For one thing, Stevenson knew that Mario's private nature and quietness were interpreted by some as standoffishness. The coach counseled the player to pay more attention to being courteous to people, and, as Lemieux would later remember, "He wanted me to be polite with the older people, with the parents and people surrounding me. He said you should respect others and I think I learned that."

For Mario, hockey was first and foremost in his life— and his parents supported him all the way, even if it meant that school took a secondary role. In fact, his parents allowed him to sleep late whenever he pleased, and with so many games and practices each season, he was often tired. His attendance at school was sporadic, but his teachers, well aware that Mario was destined for a great career in hockey, gave him passing grades nevertheless.

At 16, Mario entered the midget level and played for a new, relatively weak team, Concordia. He led his league in scoring with 62 goals in 40 games (a midget scoring

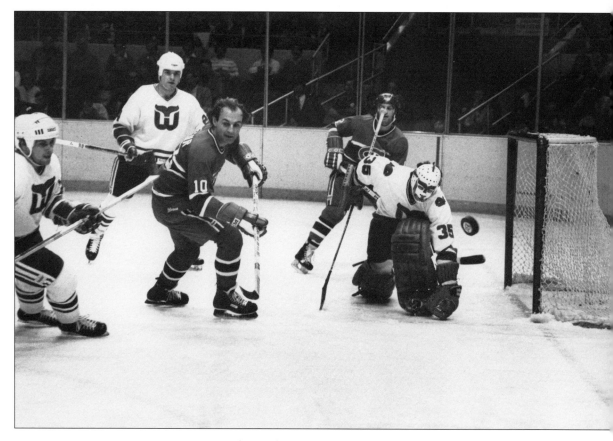

Hockey star Guy Lafleur, who played for the Canadiens, was Mario's idol throughout the 1970s. Honored as Montreal's youth player of the month when he was 12, Mario was allowed to sit behind the Canadiens' bench and see Lafleur score his 500th goal. This picture of Lafleur (center) was taken in December 1981.

record), and even tallied an overtime goal in a playoff game with a bad cut on his hand. Now it was time to move up to the next level—junior hockey—the launching pad for a professional career.

Canadian junior hockey is a peculiar institution. It is based on the old apprenticeship system—the idea being that young men learn a trade by working at the job, and earn experience rather than money. Thus in junior hockey, boys between the ages of 16 and 20 play in a league that is just like a professional hockey league in every aspect—except the players do not get paid. They are drafted and then must go to the team that selects them, even if that team is hundreds of miles from their home. They play a 70-game regular-season schedule plus the playoffs, which requires thousands upon thousands of miles of bus travel, often in the dead of the northern winter. They can be traded from one team to another at any time, or even dismissed altogether.

For all this work, the junior players' only compensation is a small daily stipend for meals, free boarding with a family that houses them, some tutoring whenever possible, and the hope that an NHL team will draft them and reward them with a big contract when it is time.

This is what the young Mario Lemieux faced after his year with Concordia. And he looked forward to it eagerly.

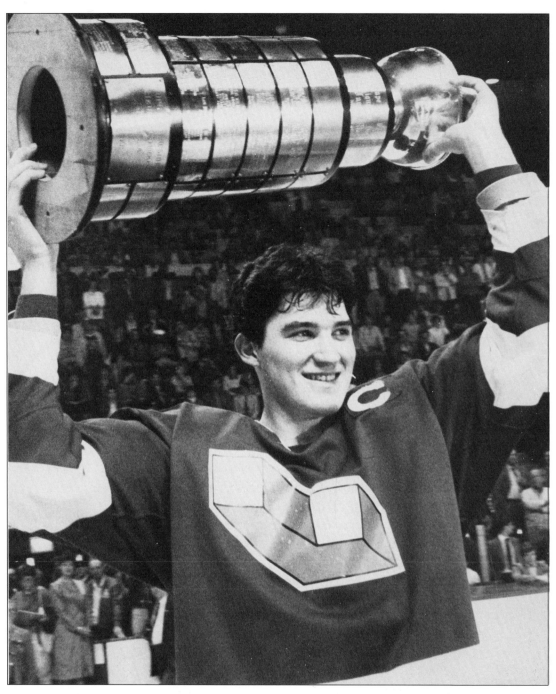

In his last year as a junior player (1983–84), Mario led the Laval Voisins to the Quebec Major Junior Hockey League (QMJHL) title.

4

THE JOURNEY
THROUGH JUNIORS

MARIO LEMIEUX was the first player picked in the Quebec Major
Junior Hockey League (QMJHL) midget draft for the 1981–82 season.
In hockey, as in other North American sports, the team that finishes
last the previous season is able to select first in the draft. Mario was
chosen by the Laval Voisins, located just outside Montreal (*voisins* is
the French word for "neighbors"). Mario promptly promised the Laval
owner that the Voisins would win the Memorial Cup, emblematic of
the Canadian national junior championship, during his junior career.

   Prior to the draft, Mario had been contacted by Bob Perno, an agent
who worked with Gus Badali, Wayne Gretzky's agent. Gretzky, entering his second year in the NHL, was already being hailed as the greatest
hockey player who ever lived—greater even than Bobby Orr, Gordie
Howe, or Maurice Richard. He was born and raised in Brantford,
Ontario, and learned to skate at age two and a half in a backyard rink

Wayne Gretzky, nicknamed the Great One, is perhaps the greatest hockey player of all time. He was starting his second year with the National Hockey League (NHL) when Mario was drafted in the QMJHL. The two hockey players had met and Gretzky became Mario's mentor of sorts.

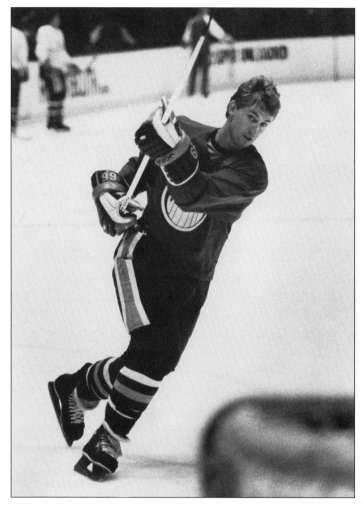

made by his father. At six years old Gretzky was already well known across Canada, and at age 10 he astounded the nation by tallying 378 goals in 85 games. At 17 he turned professional with the Indianapolis Racers of the World Hockey Association (WHA), a short-lived rival league of the NHL, and when that team started to run out of money he was sold to another WHA club, the Edmonton Oilers. Gretzky went on to score 46 goals and 64 assists for 110 points in his rookie season, which also happened to be the final year for the WHA. He was the WHA's number three scorer that year, and number one on a points-per-game basis.

The next season, 1979–80, the Oilers were absorbed into the NHL and the adolescent Gretzky shocked everyone by tallying 137 points with 51 goals and 86 assists, missing the scoring title by an eyelash. But Gretzky did become the youngest player ever to score 50 goals in a season, and he had served notice that there was simply no limit to what he could do in his career. In 1980–81, the year Mario spent with Concordia, Gretzky ran away with the NHL scoring title, racking up 164 points, a record 109 of them coming from assists. And he had just turned 20 years old.

The boyishly charming and unfailingly polite Gretzky, already nicknamed the Great One, was immensely popular throughout Canada. He appeared in advertisements for various products, for which he was paid handsomely, augmenting his already lucrative contract with the Oilers.

Mario felt he was headed in the same direction, so he listened closely when Perno approached him and his family about becoming his agent. The key question that Mario had for Perno was, simply, how much money could he get for his first NHL contract three years down the road? Perno replied by saying a million dollars, at which point Mario announced that Perno would be his agent.

In August 1981, Mario Lemieux, accompanied by Perno, met Wayne Gretzky for the first time at a charity golf tournament in Toronto. The Great One invited Mario to come watch the shooting of a TV commercial he would be in, and Mario obliged. Afterward, Gretzky invited him out for dinner, followed by drinks—despite Mario's tender age—at a disco on Yonge Street, one of Toronto's nightlife districts. Even though Mario did not speak English very well at the time, he listened as Gretzky offered advice on all the things Mario was sure to encounter in the years ahead—contracts, endorsements, who might help him, who to watch out for, and so on.

There was more excitement in store for Mario that evening. As Lawrence Martin writes:

> [Gretzky] fell into conversation with a couple of adoring girls, both of whom knew of him, of course, but not of his friend Mario. Continuing his performance as the perfect host, Gretzky introduced one of the girls to Mario. The four of them then adjourned to the Westbury Hotel, where they spent the night and, if what Mario later told a friend was true, a big moment in his young life took place.

Given that Mario Lemieux would one day be considered the only player who could challenge Wayne Gretzky as the game's top player, the historic implications of what happened that night are mind-boggling. But in any case, perhaps as a result of his evening with Gretzky, Lemieux told Perno that he would like to change his sweater number when he started playing for Laval that fall, from his usual 27 to Gretzky's 99 (until the mid-1970s, few hockey players wore numbers above 35). Perno thought that in a sense the number 99 belonged exclusively to Gretzky; that for anyone else to wear the number would be an act of arrogance. In the end, they settled on another distinctive number: 66. It would come to be associated with Mario Lemieux, and years later no young hockey phenom would dare wear that number for precisely the same reason Mario did not wear number 99.

Mario was lucky to be playing for a team located so close to his home. In the Western Junior League, for example, a 16-year-old player might grow up in Vancouver on the shores of the Pacific Ocean, then be forced to play for a team in Manitoba, some 1,200 miles to the east. Mario was playing only a few miles from his home and the family to whom he was so close. Nevertheless, the Voisins' schedule and the starting times of games were such that he often had to stay at a Laval boardinghouse rather than the family home.

Mario's first year in the juniors was excellent, but he did not quite produce at the same spectacular pace he was

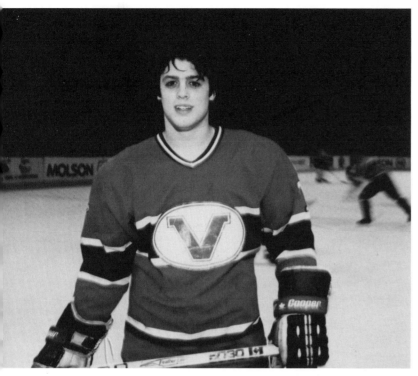

American Pat LaFontaine won the scoring award over Mario Lemieux in the QMJHL 1982–83 season. Although Mario lost the scoring race, he led Laval to a first-place regular-season finish.

used to. He scored 30 goals and 66 assists in 60 regular-season games, helping Laval to a 7th-place finish—a marked improvement over the 10th-place final standing of the previous year. He added another 5 goals and 9 assists in 18 playoff contests—totals that were good enough to lead all QMJHL rookies. But given the grand expectations for Mario, some writers labeled his performance as disappointing. In the end, he just missed getting the league's rookie of the year award, which surprised and frustrated him and his family. After the season was over, Mario decided that he would devote all his energy to hockey.

Thus, at age 16 and on his way to entering 11th grade, he decided to drop out of school. His family agreed with his decision without raising a fuss, because a professional hockey career was what Mario was definitely headed for, and they believed he should concentrate on getting there. Perno and Badali compensated somewhat by signing

Mario up for English courses, so that he would be fluent in the language by the time he made it to the NHL.

The following season Mario blossomed as a player. Already big enough to handle himself in any of the blood-curdling brawls that mark junior hockey, as players try to impress professional scouts and one another with their toughness, Mario regained the full extent of his magnificent scoring touch. He propelled the Voisins to first place through the first two and a half months of the season. But to his surprise, he had company at the top—an American named Pat LaFontaine from the Detroit, Michigan, area.

Small, fast, charismatic, and in his last eligible year of the juniors, LaFontaine was a popular player—perhaps because of his French Canadian ancestry or the eagerness with which he, an Anglophone, studied the French language. But LaFontaine was also red hot, and by mid-December he had opened up a big lead on Mario atop the scoring charts. Mario had been chosen to be on the Canadian national team for the 1982 world junior championships, to be held that year in Leningrad in the Soviet Union. Just before Christmas, he left Laval and the scoring race behind and joined the national team for the two-week tournament.

In modern hockey, most teams play with four lines; that is, four trios consisting of a left wing, center, and right wing. The first line gets the most ice time and is expected to do much of the scoring; being a first-line center was Mario's accustomed role. The second line does not get as much ice time as the first, but it too is expected to score a lot. The third line is usually referred to as the checking line; its job is to thwart the other team's first line. Finally there is the fourth line, which sees very little ice; its main job is to give everyone else a rest.

In Leningrad, the Canadian coach, Dave King, stressed a defensive, close-checking game. He believed that Mario paid too little attention to *back-checking* and other defensive aspects of play, and relegated him to the little-used fourth line. After seeing spot duty during the first three games of the tournament, Mario was benched outright, then put back on the fourth line. To make matters worse, he suffered a slight knee injury. Yet despite the limited play, frustration, benching, and aches and pains, Mario still scored five goals and five assists in 10 games to wind up Canada's number two scorer in the tourney. The whole Leningrad experience had been a wretched one for Mario (the last straw was Canada's disappointing third-place finish), and it soured him on the idea of international competition. In future years, he would often turn down invitations to play for Canada, drawing the ire of his countrymen.

When he got back to Laval, Mario found that LaFontaine had an insurmountable lead in the scoring race. He also found the Voisins out of first place and falling fast, so if he could do nothing about catching the American, he could at least do something about rescuing his team. Scoring at a pace of better than three points per game, Mario not only stopped the Voisins' slide but got the team to improve its standing. They finished the regular season in first place. Mario ranked number two in the QMJHL with 84 goals and 100 assists in 66 games, and was named the league's second team all-star center. He added a remarkable 32 points in 12 playoff games, but the Voisins fell before reaching the league final. Mario had one more year of juniors left before the NHL draft. But if his third year with Laval resembled the first two, he probably would not be able to attract the million-dollar professional contract he hoped to sign. To get the big money, he knew he would have to make his final amateur year an unforgettable one.

He got the 1983–84 season off to an incredible start, scoring 35 points in his first seven games. It was clear that Mario had a shot at two cherished QMJHL single-season records: Guy Lafleur's 130 goals in 1971 and Pierre Larouche's 251 points in 1974. By the middle of Novem-

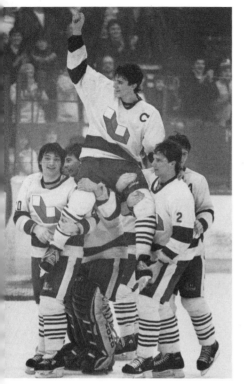

After breaking Guy Lafleur's QMJHL record of 130 goals in a single season, Mario is carried off the ice by his teammates in the last game of the 1983–84 season. Before the game, Mario had called it "the biggest match I will play since I have put on skates."

ber, Mario was up to 101 points in 25 games, and the Voisins had won 20 games, tied 2, and lost only 3. At this point, the controversy surrounding the world junior championships arose again.

The Canadian team wanted Mario to join them once again for the tournament, which would be played in Sweden in December. But he refused. The previous year's experience, he said, had been too unpleasant. He also wanted to stay with the Voisins to help it advance to the league and even the national championships. Finally, there was the important matter of trying to break Lafleur and Larouche's records. The QMJHL executive board tried to persuade Mario to play for Canada, threatening to suspend him if he continued to refuse, but he held firm. As biographer Lawrence Martin observed, "They didn't know Lemieux. The streak of stubbornness that ran through him was a steel cord. 'If somebody yells at me to hurry up,' Mario said once in a comment that always applied, 'I slow down.' "

The league announced that Mario would be suspended for four games—the same number of games he would have missed had he gone to Sweden to play for the national team. Mario and Perno responded quickly and forcefully. They hired a lawyer and challenged the QMJHL's suspension in Quebec superior court. Shortly thereafter the court handed down its decision: there was nothing in Mario Lemieux's contract with the Laval Voisins or the QMJHL to force him to play for Canada. He was free to refuse the national team's invitation. Mario returned to action for Laval without having missed a single game, and he continued to score at a record pace.

But many in the hockey establishment and the hockey media were souring on him because of the world junior championship controversy. Some called him unpatriotic for refusing to represent his country. In Canada, such accusations are sometimes loaded in a way that people in some other countries might find hard to understand.

French-language newspapers in Quebec generally sided with Mario, pointing out that the coaches of the Canadian junior team were English speaking, both in 1982 (Dave King) and 1983 (Brian Kilrea). They suggested that perhaps Mario had been benched by King because Mario was a Francophone. Furthermore, some pointed out, there were usually a disproportionately small number of French Canadians on national junior teams because, they argued, it was English Canadians who usually chose the players for international play. To his credit, Mario denied that Canada's 300-year-old rift between French and English had anything to do with his decision not to play in the tournament.

Mario cruised through the winter and took dead aim at the scoring records. With five games left in the season, he passed Larouche's 251 points. Going into the final game, a home contest, he needed three goals to tie Lafleur's mark of 130. It just so happened that Gretzky's team, the Edmonton Oilers, were in Montreal to play the Habs that night. Perno brought Gretzky to the Laval game to see whether Mario could break the record. It took just 43 seconds for Mario to score his first goal, and another 80 seconds to score his second. A little over a minute into the middle period, he scored again to tie Lafleur at 130. When he notched his fourth goal of the evening six minutes later, the record was his. He added two more goals that night, and Gretzky saw it all.

Mario wound up with mind-boggling season totals of 133 goals and 149 assists for 282 points. Ten years later, when Mario Lemieux announced that he had Hodgkin's disease, the goals and points he made in that game would still be all-time Canadian junior records. But no matter how well any player or team does in the regular season, in hockey success and failure are measured by performance in the playoffs. Mario had promised that Laval would win the Memorial Cup for Canada's junior championship, but in order to do that, the Voisins would first have to win the QMJHL playoffs.

This they did, with Mario leading the way by collecting a record 29 goals and 23 assists in only 14 postseason games. Laval had reached the Memorial Cup, which was being played that year in Kitchener, Ontario. The Memorial Cup tournament pitted the winners of Canada's three major junior leagues (the Quebec, Ontario, and Western leagues) plus the team from the host city against each other, with the winner being crowned Canada's junior champion. Suddenly, everything shiny and magical for Mario and the Voisins crumbled to dust in the opener against Kitchener. Mario was held scoreless for only the second time in the season as Laval fell 8–2. Laval's coach accused Mario of laziness, and Mario replied that the coach had "better keep his mouth shut."

Mario Lemieux was named the QMJHL most valuable player for the 1983–84 season, tallying goals and assists that are junior league records to this day and finishing his junior career with the best three-season record in the history of Quebec.

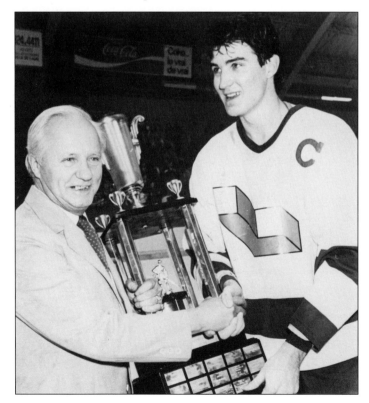

The second game, against the Ontario champs from Ottawa, went a bit better, but Laval lost again, 6–5. When they lost their third game 4–3 to the Western champ, Kamloops, it was all over. Three games, three losses, and a humiliating elimination. Lemieux had scored only three points. "It was as close as he ever came to failure," Perno later told Jean Sonmor. "I remember those nights after the games, the long postmortems with his parents. I don't think Mario knew what was wrong. He'd played nearly 100 games at a supernatural pace; maybe he was just worn out."

The defeat in the Memorial Cup made some observers wonder whether Mario had what it takes to be a champion. It was fairly well known among NHL general managers and some hockey writers that Mario liked to sleep a lot, that he smoked cigarettes (a habit he had started at age 16), that he ate a lot of junk food, and that he did not like to exercise or lift weights. He had seemed to sulk when Dave King had put him on the fourth line for the 1982 world junior championships, and he defied the QMJHL and national team authorities by taking them to court the following year.

Despite all the records and the vastly improved play of his team, did Mario have an attitude problem that would prevent him from achieving ultimate success in the NHL?

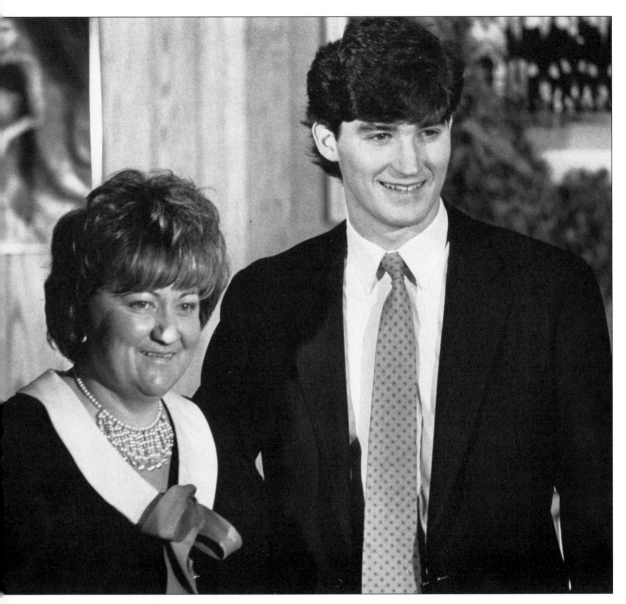

When the Pittsburgh Penguins chose Mario Lemieux in the 1984 National Hockey League draft, Lemieux refused to accept the contract that the team offered him. A week after the draft, the two sides made an agreement. Two years later, Lemieux had proved himself to be one of the greatest hockey players of all time, and he signed a contract that made him the second highest-paid player in the NHL. Lemieux and his mother are seen here in 1986, after Lemieux's signing of the new five-year contract.

5

THE FLIGHTLESS BIRDS

EVERY HOCKEY FAN ON THE CONTINENT knew that Mario Lemieux was going to be the first player chosen in the draft for the 1984–85 NHL season. And that meant he would be picked by the Pittsburgh Penguins, the last-place team in the league the previous year. The Montreal Canadiens had tried to be in position to draft Lemieux. Two years before, they traded one of their young stars to the lowly Hartford Whalers in order to get the Whalers' position in the 1984 draft, where they hoped to choose Lemieux. But alas, the Whalers were not quite as bad as Pittsburgh, and the Penguins earned the number one pick. This suited Lemieux just fine. If most Montreal boys, including those who had made it big in junior hockey, dreamed of playing for the Canadiens, Lemieux was different. He actually preferred not to play in Montreal.

"I think it will be better for me to go to the United States," he said before the draft. "I'm not so known and there won't be so much expectation. I think it will be better for my career." Given Lemieux's very private nature, it is not surprising that he would rather play far from hockey's limelight. And Pittsburgh certainly was that.

The NHL had been a six-team league since the World War II era, with teams in Montreal, Toronto, Boston, Detroit, New York, and Chicago. In 1967 it expanded to six new cities, one of which was Pittsburgh. The Penguins did not get off to a strong start, losing often in their first years. In 1969–70, a French Canadian named Michel Brière had a promising rookie season for the Penguins, but he died of injuries sustained in an automobile accident during the off-season. In 1974–75 another French Canadian rookie, Pierre Larouche, who had set the QMJHL point record that Lemieux would break a few years later, helped lead the Penguins to their first-ever winning season. But that year the team became only the second in NHL history to blow a three games to zero lead and lose a playoff series. The team promptly declared bankruptcy. New owners rescued the Penguins, but through the next few years their record dropped down to the .500 level and below.

During an intermission in one game, Penguins player Brian "Spinner" Spencer appeared as a guest on the game telecast, declared that the team's problems stemmed from its name ("Whoever heard of a team named after a *penguin?*"), then proceeded to smash up the set.

In 1983, the team's general manager, Baz Bastien, died in an automobile accident, adding another sad chapter to the team's woebegone history. Bastien's successor as Pittsburgh's general manager was Eddie Johnston, and some say that in the season prior to the NHL draft in which Lemieux was available, he did all he could to ensure that the Penguins would finish last. Whether this is true is debatable, but it is a fact that the Penguins finished the 1983–84 season with the worst record in franchise history.

The Penguins management saw the imminent arrival of Lemieux as a godsend. Here, they thought, was the player who would lead the team out of the doldrums and into the upper reaches of the standings. Here, they believed, was a player so exciting to watch that he would draw more than the paltry average of under 7,000 fans who attended games at Pittsburgh's Civic Arena, nicknamed the Igloo for its domelike shape. Fired with enthusiasm, the Penguins started distributing brochures hailing the arrival of the big teenage superstar, hoping to convince more Pittsburghers to buy season tickets. There was only one catch: Lemieux had not yet been drafted by the Penguins—he had certainly not signed with them, and he had never given permission for the team to use his name to sell tickets.

An angry Lemieux, who through Perno had been talking with the Penguins about what salary he would receive for signing with the club, told the *Toronto Sun,* "It's hard to negotiate when they want you for nothing and you want the big bucks."

As draft day approached, the two sides could not agree on the terms of a contract. Despite the friction, the Penguins were so optimistic about Lemieux that they sold tickets to fans so they could view the draft proceedings on a giant TV screen as they were beamed in from Montreal. And so desperate were Penguins fans for a winner that 4,000 of them showed up to watch.

Although Lemieux was still fuming about the contract impasse, he came to the draft at the Montreal Forum anyway. But when Johnston announced that the Penguins had selected Mario Lemieux as the number one pick, Lemieux stayed in his seat. Johnston repeated himself, but again Lemieux refused to acknowledge him. As reporters and photographers gathered around, they found Pierrette crying. Lemieux briefly rose, waved for a moment, then sat down again. Both in the Forum and several hundred miles away at the Igloo, fans were aghast. What was going on? A Penguins team official came over to where Lemieux,

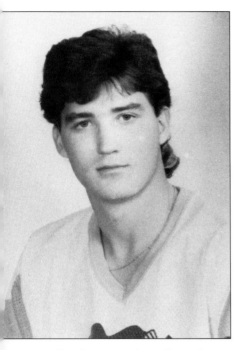

Lemieux, wearing a Penguins jersey, poses for a headshot before his rookie season in 1984.

his family, and his agents were sitting, but left after a brief argument. While other draftees went up to shake hands with the general managers who had drafted them and don the sweaters of their new teams, Lemieux and his party went nowhere—except, eventually, out of the Forum.

Predictably, Canada's English-language hockey media criticized Lemieux, while the French-language media supported him. "I'm a francophone and the draft is in Quebec and I'm not afraid to stand up to them," he told the French-language newspapers.

But the storm blew over quickly. Within a week, Lemieux signed a contract worth somewhere between $600,000 and $750,000 for two years, with bonuses that brought the final total as high as $900,000—not quite the million dollar pact he had dreamed of, but still the richest rookie contract in NHL history. When *Sports Illustrated* asked Lemieux a few months later about what happened on draft day, he replied, "I don't regret doing that. One week later I had my contract." Besides, at his first press conference soon after arriving in Pittsburgh, he put on a Penguins sweater after all.

Lemieux had to move away from his close-knit family and the country where he lived his entire life and move to the United States, where he would not even be comfortable speaking the language. (He later said that he learned English by watching soap operas.) He was only 18 years old, so Perno decided the adjustment would be easier for Lemieux if he boarded with a family rather than try to manage a home of his own. Lemieux wound up living with the well-off Mathews family in their large house in the Pittsburgh suburb of Mount Lebanon, a place he would soon call his second home.

In mid-September 1984, the Penguins' training camp opened at the Mount Lebanon Ice Arena. Lemieux, in his first intrasquad game wearing the black, gold, and white colors of the Penguins, impressed everyone present. "Mario did some great things out there today—scary things," Pittsburgh scout Bruce Haralson told *Sports Illustrated.* "He did things only Gretzky can do. That's what's scary—to think that there might be another one." Scarier still was the fact that Lemieux did miserably in all the strength tests and was unable to keep up with anyone else on the team while jogging—yet he was still the best player in camp.

October 11 was the night of the Penguins' season opener and Lemieux's NHL debut against the Boston Bruins at the cramped old Boston Garden. Coming onto the ice in the second minute of play, Lemieux intercepted an errant pass at center ice, barged in all alone on a *breakaway,* shifted the puck from forehand to backhand, deking Bruins goalkeeper Pete Peeters out of the play, and shoveling the puck into the open net for a goal. Quite a debut, even if the Penguins lost. "I stood in there, forced him to make a move, and he made a move," said Peeters after the game. "The thing I forgot was that he's got that great reach."

The second game, in the famed Montreal Forum itself, was also a loss. Lemieux did not do much in that game, but he did receive a warm reception from his old hometown fans.

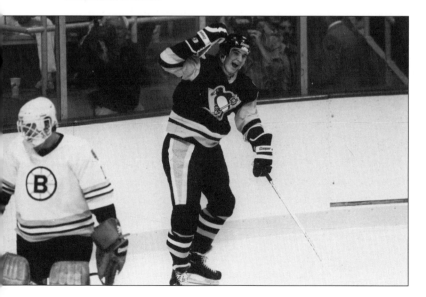

Lemieux celebrates his first NHL goal, scored against the Bruins at the Boston Garden at the beginning of the first period.

The third game was Pittsburgh's Civic Arena opener, before Lemieux's new hometown fans. A near sellout crowd of 15,000 turned out for the game against Vancouver, and in the first 18 seconds they saw Lemieux set up a teammate for a goal. On his second shift, they saw him

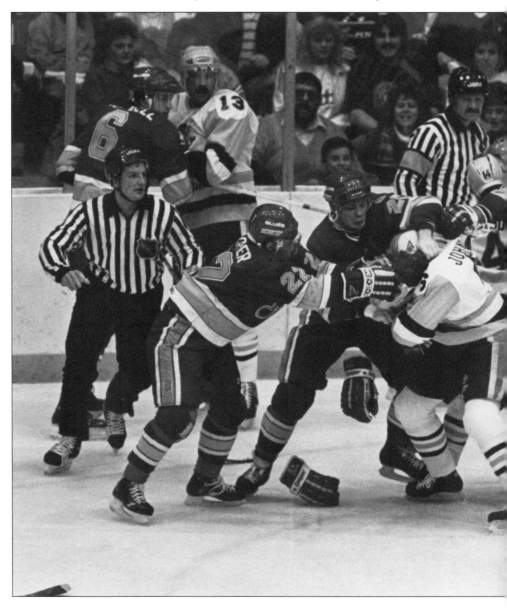

square off for a fight with a Canuck player named Gary Lupul. Fighting, of course, is tolerated in the juniors and in the NHL, and some players base their entire career on being able to fight whenever and wherever called for. Other players fight occasionally, some as a deliberate

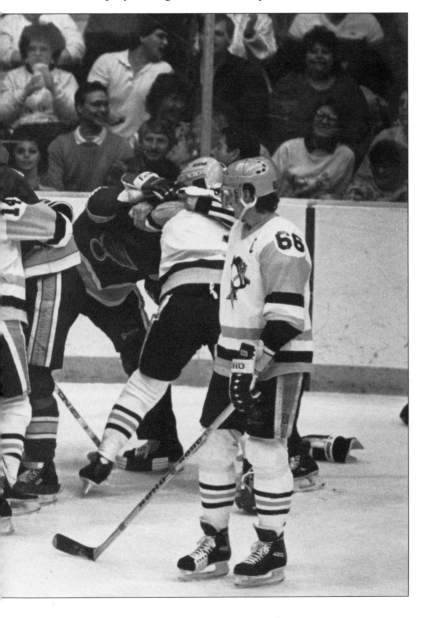

Lemieux (far right) looks on while his teammates fight the St. Louis Blues. Not much of a fighter, Lemieux had a bout with a Canuck player in one of his first NHL games, but throughout the years he rarely fought again.

tactic intended to intimidate the other team, some out of genuine spontaneous anger. Some players progress through their entire career without dropping the gloves—but often a much-heralded rookie, even if he is not the fighting type, must prove himself early on by mixing it up with an opponent. The one fight in the entire 17-year NHL career of the great Quebecois and Buffalo Sabres star Gil Perreault took place in one of the first NHL games he played; he thrashed a Los Angeles tough guy named Dan Maloney and was never challenged again.

Such was the case with Lemieux. He tangled with Lupul and pummeled him, forcing the Canuck to do what in hockey parlance is called turtling up—dropping face-down to the ice and covering up so that only the back is exposed to the blows raining down on a player. Lemieux skated off to the penalty box to the cheers of the Igloo crowd. He was having a good debut with the Penguins. Pittsburgh coach Bob Berry enthused, "No one who's come out of junior hockey has ever shown as much potential as Mario—ever."

That start was derailed briefly by a knee injury that kept him out of seven games, but when he returned he started a scoring streak. By mid-January 1985 he had registered 21 goals and 35 assists in 42 games—far better than the point-per-game pace that in the high-scoring 1980s marked the difference between excellent veterans and journeymen. What was all the more remarkable was that Lemieux was a rookie and was on pace to chase some records of first-year players.

Nevertheless, there were questions about Lemieux's back-checking; that is, his defensive game. Indeed, he would finish the season with a poor defensive record, with a rating of minus 35. (In hockey, statistics are kept to measure each player's defensive ability by tallying the number of even-strength goals that are scored by the player's team and those scored by the opposing team while the player is on the ice. Therefore, Lemieux's rating of minus 35 means that the opposing teams scored 35 more goals than the Penguins did while he was on the ice.) Never a very physical player in the sense of running into opponents to dislodge the puck from them or simply to rattle them, he also was not the type of player to come back into his own zone to help prevent goals. Lemieux figured his job was to score goals, or at least to set up goals. And as to charges that he did not try very hard while on the ice, he always countered that it only looked that way, that he was actually playing quite hard but his size and long, loping stride made it look like he was lazy.

"Hockey Night in Canada" commentator Don Cherry, the most ebullient and controversial hockey critic on the continent, disagreed. Cherry called Lemieux "the biggest floater in the league," a reputation that Lemieux already had, and one that would haunt him until he announced that he had Hodgkin's disease. Soon after Cherry's pronouncement, Lemieux was selected for the annual NHL all-star game, where he faced off against Gretzky and the rest of the league's top stars. And the big rookie sparkled, scoring two goals and an assist to earn Most Valuable Player (MVP) honors. Along with the award for his superb playing, he won a new truck, which he gave to his brother Richard.

Lemieux continued to score throughout the rest of the season, and even though the Penguins' performance was still unsatisfactory (they finished with an awful 24 wins, 51 losses, and 5 ties, which was actually a substantial improvement over the previous season), he racked up some impressive individual achievements. In 73 games he scored 43 goals and 57 assists for 100 points—the third highest total for any rookie in league history (behind Peter Stastny of the Quebec Nordiques, who scored 109 points in 1981, and Dale Hawerchuk of the Winnipeg Jets, who scored 103 points in 1982). He won the 1985 Calder Trophy as rookie of the year. Also during his premiere year, he set up his linemate, 30-year-old career minor leaguer Warren Young, in his first NHL season, for 40 goals. Young parlayed this success into a big contract with Detroit for his final pro years and, as he readily acknowledged, he owed it to Lemieux. Last but not least, average attendance at the Civic Arena rose to 10,000.

Lemieux would have liked to go home at the end of the season, but he was persuaded to go to Prague, Czechoslovakia, for the world championships, which meant little to Canadians because they always took place during the much more prestigious Stanley Cup playoffs. The tournament also meant little to Lemieux, who still soured at the memory of his experiences at the world junior championships. When he finally got to Prague, he had to sit out a couple of games with an injury and considered going

Number 66 faces off against number 99. Comparisons between Lemieux and Wayne Gretzky had graced the sports pages and dominated conversations among hockey fans long before Lemieux began his professional career.

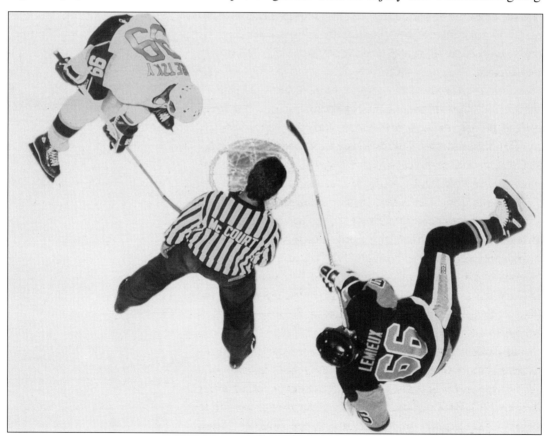

home; in the end, he stayed and starred in a 3–1 win over the Soviet Union. Canada won a silver medal with Lemieux as one of the top performers on the national team. When he returned to Ville Emard, his family threw a huge party.

Before his second season in Pittsburgh, Lemieux decided to move out of the Mathews's house and into a nearby apartment of his own. He was joined by his girlfriend, Nathalie Asselin, whom he had started going out with in Ville Emard when he was 17 and she was 15. Introduced by cousins, she had instantly fallen for him. "After the first minute, I knew," she would later recall.

Tall and athletic (she was a lifeguard when she met Mario), Asselin was 18 and spoke little English when she moved in with Lemieux. "He'd be lost without her," a Penguins player told *Sports Illustrated.* "She screens his calls, cooks for him, she's his best friend. He'd be lost, believe me."

Lemieux had further support from Nancy Mathews, who, according to the young superstar, "still comes over all the time, cleans, brings over food. And she does my mail." The Mathews's three sons would come over to play street hockey, re-creating, at least to some degree, the warm family atmosphere experienced on rue Jorgue.

Lemieux also spent the summer indulging his passion for golf. He had been introduced to the game at age 15 by Bob Perno, and in his first outing had shot a 116 for 18 holes—an impressive but not overly remarkable debut. However, after a few more times out he was breaking 100, and within a year, he had gotten his score down into the 80s—something many golfers spend their whole lives trying to do.

Golf would prove to be Lemieux's one off-ice enthusiasm, his one true extracurricular activity. During off-seasons, training camps, or stops in warm-weather cities during the NHL season, Lemieux would always take time to play a round or two. Especially in the summer, when there are numerous charity golf tournaments, Lemieux could be found on the links with other hockey players, who are famed for their love of golf.

Lemieux, however, was special. His golf game was so excellent that many believed he would try to join the professional tour upon his retirement. And in later years, when the specter of cancer and other maladies would come to haunt him, many feared that this very retirement would come far too early.

If there was any doubt that Lemieux warranted all the comparisons to Gretzky, they were dispelled in his sophomore season, 1985–86. By January, he was second in scoring in the entire NHL only to Gretzky himself. When the Penguins went to Edmonton to play the Oilers, Lemieux came out on top, scoring a goal and three assists to Gretzky's two assists in a 7–4 win. By the season's three-quarter mark, Lemieux had notched a fabulous 38 goals and 72 assists for 110 points. The Great One, however, had 164 points. Even though some were touting Lemieux as the imminent heir apparent to Gretzky's mantle as the world's greatest player, he clearly had far to go. Gretzky said of Lemieux, "Maybe he'll give me a push one of these seasons." Lemieux agreed, saying, "I'm not at the same level as Gretzky yet."

It was also true that Gretzky played alongside excellent teammates, a luxury Lemieux did not have. The Penguins, however, were improving, playing at just over a .500 clip. Still reserved, Lemieux revealed little about himself, but details were starting to emerge. When Bob Kravitz of *Sports Illustrated* visited Lemieux's apartment in his second season, he found that Lemieux did "a better-than-average impersonation of Elvis Presley and an equally good, but more improbable one, of Pee-Wee Herman."

His teammate and road roommate Terry Ruskowski observed, "Nobody sleeps as well as Mario. He lives for sleep. He hits the bed and that's it. It irritates the hell out of me."

Perno noted about the young star's personality:

Around the people he doesn't really know or people in the hockey world—teammates and reporters—he has an image he must project. And knows that. Always smiling, taking things in stride. He has unbelievable maturity in that sense, a 20-year-old going on 28.

But when you get him away from that scene, get him back home with friends, he reverts to being an 18-year-old. I remember the night before we signed his new contract this winter. There was still a lot of pressure. I was nervous, his dad was nervous. So we're sitting there in his apartment and Mario says, "Let's play Intellivision Football [a video game]." I swear, he was more interested in beating me at Intellivision Football than he was about a multimillion-dollar contract.

In February, Lemieux sat out a game with the back problems that had first flared up in the juniors and would plague him for the rest of his career. When he returned, the Penguins were still in the hunt for a playoff spot. But they went into a tailspin, losing 12 of their last 16 games—including 1 to Edmonton in which Gretzky outscored Lemieux four to one. The Penguins wound up four games below .500 and missed the playoffs. It was a disappointing finish, but the average number of spectators was now over 11,000. The continued rise in attendance allayed fears that the team might have to move to another city. It was said that Lemieux saved hockey in Pittsburgh.

As for Lemieux himself, he ended up with a whopping 48 goals and 93 assists for 141 points, one of the highest totals in NHL history. Wayne Gretzky won the scoring title that year, however, with an astounding 52 goals and 163 assists for 215 points. Those assists and points totals are all-time NHL records. Already, Lemieux was being called the second-best player in the world. And now he had a nickname of his own, Mario *le Magnifique*—Mario *the Magnificent*.

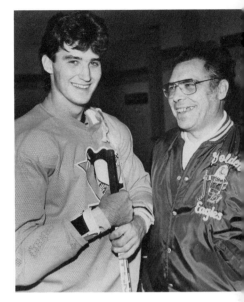

Jean-Guy Lemieux stands next to his favorite hockey player—his son Mario—in 1985. A proud father, Jean-Guy had been an avid hockey fan his entire life and pushed Mario to be the best he could be.

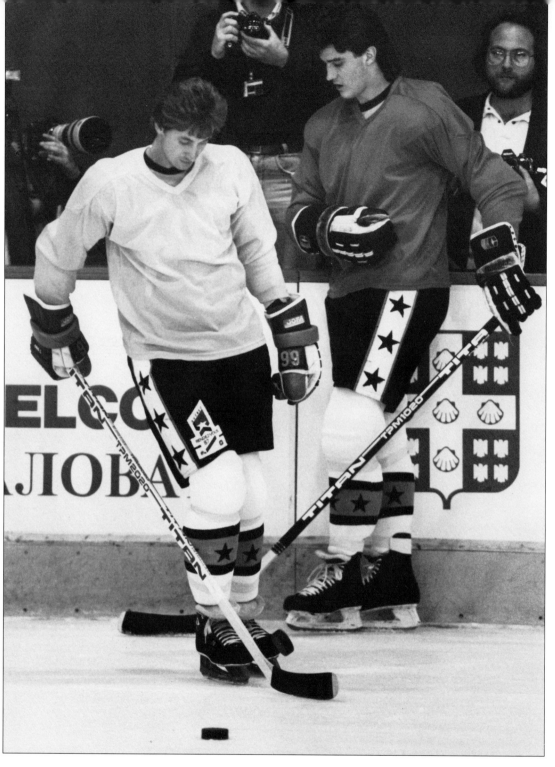

Lemieux (right) and Gretzky practice before the Canada Cup tournament in February 1987. Two of hockey's greatest players skating on the same team were too much to handle for the Soviet team, which went down in defeat.

6

THE LONG
ASCENT BEGINS

THE 1986–87 SEASON, Lemieux's third in Pittsburgh, started with a seven-game winning streak before settling back into the usual .500 rut. In late December, Lemieux was out with a bad knee, and by now everyone had pretty much gotten the idea that Lemieux was injury prone. Soon after his return, he got into a fight with a Washington player named Bobby Gould, who knocked Lemieux unconscious. It was not the first time he had been the victim of a punch-out, but it was the only time thus far that he had really been hurt.

In any case, his triumph in the first professional fight of his rookie year was a distant memory now. The Penguins were still a weak team. They continued their ineffectual play, despite Lemieux's big-point totals, and finished eight games below .500, missing the playoffs once again. Playing in only 63 games, Lemieux had his first 50-goal season, finishing with 54 goals, 53 assists, and 107 points, the third best in the NHL.

For the second straight year, Lemieux refused to play in the year-end world championships in Europe. Hockey people openly questioned his intensity, his dedication to his team, and his commitment to hockey. But if the annual world championships held little interest for the North American hockey world, another tourney, the quadrennial Canada Cup tournament, held plenty.

Every four years the best performers from the top-six hockey-playing nations on earth assembled in September to decide which country was the best, and 1987 marked the fourth renewal of the competition. Canada and the Soviet Union were the favorites, with Czechoslovakia, Sweden, the United States, and Finland all providing stiff competition. Canada and the United States were made up entirely of NHLers, while the Scandinavians carried several and the Czechoslovaks possessed a handful. The Soviets, still under a communist government, did not allow their players to go abroad to compete in foreign leagues. Since 1972, when the Canadians and Soviets met for the first time in a special eight-game series, the international collisions between the two hockey powers swelled with drama.

In that first clash, the heavily favored Canadians were shocked by the speed and precision of the poorly equipped Soviets and lost two of the four games played in Canada. Back to Moscow for the final four games, however, and Team Canada, with hard-earned respect for their opponents, rallied to tie the series. In the final minute of the final game, Canada scored the series-winning goal— a moment no Canadian will ever forget. Yet the Soviets had served notice. In the years that followed, the Soviet Union had usually outplayed the NHLers—despite the North Americans' often brutal tactics against the Soviets, who always displayed remarkable turn-the-other-cheek restraint.

Now they would meet again, and for the first time Mario Lemieux would be there. Not only that, but he would also be teamed with Wayne Gretzky. With the tournament underway, Lemieux scored three goals against the United States and added another two plus an assist against Sweden, then garnered two goals plus an assist against Czechoslovakia. Soon the Canadians were playing in a two-out-of-three final series against the Soviet Union.

Everything that had happened before in the tournament merely served as a prelude for this final confrontation. Team Canada coach Mike Keenan did not always play Lemieux on the same line with Gretzky—for one thing, both players were centers, and both were superb *playmakers*. But when he did play them together, they shined, and people across the planet's northern tier marveled at the sight of hockey's two greatest players skating alongside each other.

"He's got those awesome wrists," said Gretzky of his temporary linemate. "He could snap a puck through a refrigerator door." Gretzky added, "We found out we weren't just friends, we were ice-mates. We understood each other."

The first game of the final set was won by the Soviets in overtime, and fans wondered whether the famous, high-paid Canadians would be upset on the international stage once again. Lemieux had two assists in defeat.

In the second game, Team Canada came back, and Lemieux was the star. He scored their last three goals, with Gretzky assisting on all of them, including the overtime winner that sent the series to a deciding game. All Canada adored Lemieux for his incredible performance in single-handedly keeping the national team alive.

The third game would go down in history as one of the greatest ever played. Far from home, before a hostile crowd of 17,000 flag-waving Canadians in Hamilton, Ontario, the Soviets built a narrow lead through their splendid weaving, counterattacking style. Team Canada fought

back, and in the final minutes the two sides were tied at
5–5. Here, the Soviets' one fatal flaw would rise up against
them: their poor defense. It had cost them their very first
clash against Canada in 1972, and it would cost them
dearly once more. With one minute to go, the red-clad
Soviets pressed in Team Canada's end, seeking the goal
that would give them the series. But the puck went to
Gretzky, who started a counterattack. In the *neutral zone,*
a Soviet defender fell down, leaving three Canadians—
including Gretzky and Lemieux—bearing down on a lone
Soviet defenseman and the goaltender. At the last moment,
Gretzky slipped a pass to Lemieux, who waited, waited,
waited—and delivered an impossible-to-stop wrist shot
over the Soviet goalie's right shoulder. Lemieux and
Gretzky embraced behind the net amid a scene of explo-
sive euphoria, as Soviet coach Viktor Tikhonov screamed
at the dejected defensemen on the bench.

In the hubbub of the locker room, the first thing said by
Gretzky, always prepared to do or say just the right thing
at the time when most others would be wrapped up in the
moment, was that he wished his grandmother a happy
birthday. He had scored 21 points, tops in the Canada Cup,
and won the tournament's most valuable player award.
Lemieux had scored 18 points, including a tourney-high
11 goals. He was hailed across Canada fors his performance, but still there was the lingering sentiment that he
was the beneficiary of Gretzky's largess.

The 1987–88 NHL regular season opened soon afterward, but it was more of the same for Pittsburgh—at least
until late November, when they acquired another superstar
to complement Lemieux. Paul Coffey had been the high-
scoring defenseman on Gretzky's Oilers since 1980. Three
times he had scored more than 100 points in a season—
only one other defenseman had scored so many in one
year—and in 1986 he had broken the single-season record
for goals by a *blueliner.* In 1984 he had finished second in
the league to Gretzky in scoring, and in 1986 was third

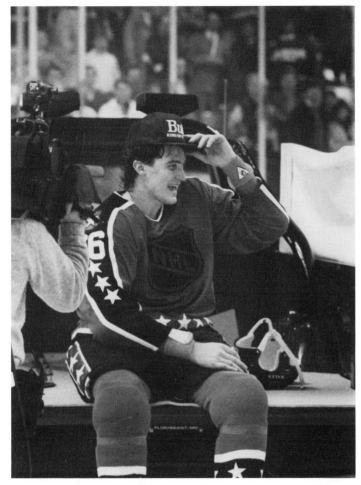

Lemieux sits on the back
of the truck that he won
after being named the most
valuable player in the 1988
All-Star Game.

behind Gretzky and Lemieux. Well on his way to breaking every career scoring mark for defenders, Coffey also had two Stanley Cup rings to show for his efforts. Now he would be coming to Pittsburgh, finally giving Lemieux someone else with extraordinary offensive skills with whom he could work.

There was more history to Coffey as well. He had been present in Laval the night Lemieux broke the junior goal-scoring record, having accompanied Gretzky to that game. Now upon arriving in Pittsburgh he inspired Lemieux and the Penguins to a modest winning streak—only to go down with a knee injury soon thereafter. Over in Edmonton, Gretzky was also injured, which left Lemieux to take over the lead for the scoring title. In the February all-star game, Lemieux was unbelievable, scoring or assisting on each one of his team's six goals, a record performance that included his winning goal in overtime. He won another truck for his achievement as all-star MVP.

He continued to sizzle throughout the rest of the season, now scoring goals at the same astounding rate that he had always helped set them up. Coffey came back late in the year and helped the Penguins' stretch run, but to no avail. Even though they finished one game above .500, they missed the playoffs. It was yet another disappointment in Lemieux's professional career. But he did finally win the

From the bench, Lemieux intently watches a play in a 1988 game. The season was a good one for Lemieux, who became only the fourth player in NHL history to score 70 goals in a season.

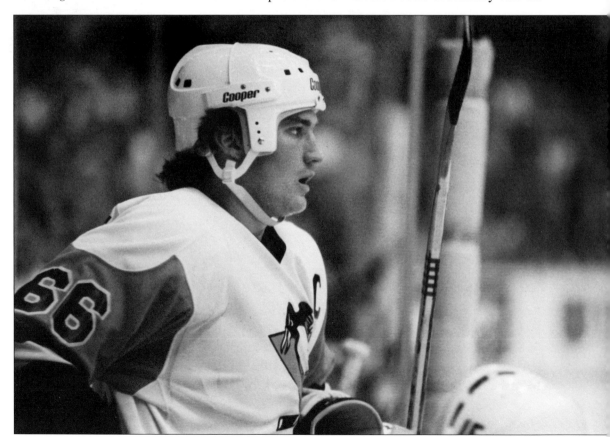

scoring title, finishing with a fantastic 70 goals and 98 assists for 168 points in 76 games. Gretzky, who had 40 goals and 109 assists for 149 points in 64 games, scored at a slightly higher per-game rate, but that did not matter. Lemieux had won the Art Ross Trophy as top scorer, breaking Gretzky's all-time record run of seven straight scoring titles. And there was more.

In 1986 Lemieux had been voted winner of the Lester B. Pearson Award, for the MVP as chosen by the NHL players themselves. Now, in 1988, he won that award again and had the satisfaction of knowing how highly his peers felt about him. But the most prestigious MVP award was still the Hart Trophy, voted on since 1924 by professional hockey writers. Gretzky had won the award an unprecedented eight times in a row—but this year the streak was broken by Lemieux.

"It started with the Canada Cup, playing with Wayne," said Lemieux. "I learned a lot from him. In my opinion, he's still the best player in the world. He had an injury this year and I took advantage of it."

In the ensuing off-season, Lemieux dropped Perno as his agent, hiring a high-powered American, Tom Reich, to take his place. Then came news that would shake the world of sports to its very foundations: Wayne Gretzky was traded to the Los Angeles Kings. Gretzky held a final news conference in Edmonton to announce that he was leaving after nine years, and broke down in tears. Canadians were shocked. How could they cope with losing Gretzky, a national treasure? And to Los Angeles, where it never snowed, where hockey was merely a cult sport followed by a few thousand people, where most citizens had never even heard of the Great One?

The real reason for the trade was financial: Oilers owner Peter Pocklington was short on cash, and received millions from the Kings as part of the deal. He also could not afford to keep paying Gretzky the millions his contract called for. However, many fans at first blamed Gretzky's new wife,

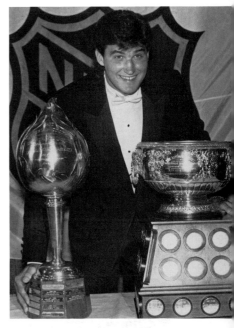

Lemieux shows off his newly won trophies for the 1987–88 season at the NHL annual awards dinner in Toronto, Canada. Lemieux won the Hart Trophy (left) for being the NHL's most valuable player and the Art Ross Trophy for winning the scoring title.

Los Angeles actress Janet Jones. They had been married just one month earlier in Edmonton in a ceremony that resembled a royal wedding. Seven hundred guests had been invited (Lemieux was not among those invited, which seemed to indicate that the Gretzky-Lemieux friendship was waning). The fans thought that Jones wanted to live in Los Angeles to stay close to her film career, but in fact this proved not to be true.

Gretzky arrived in Los Angeles to say his goal was to make hockey a big-time sport in southern California—a goal he would eventually attain. But for Lemieux, the move meant Gretzky would no longer have the supporting cast he had in Edmonton, a team that had gotten the Oilers four Stanley Cups in the previous five years.

"It's definitely going to be tougher for Gretz to reach 200 points," said Lemieux, who anticipated an easier time

Wayne Gretzky wipes tears away at a press conference announcing his trade from the Edmonton Oilers to the Los Angeles Kings. After playing for the Oilers for nine years, Gretzky said that his goal was to make hockey a big-time sport in southern California.

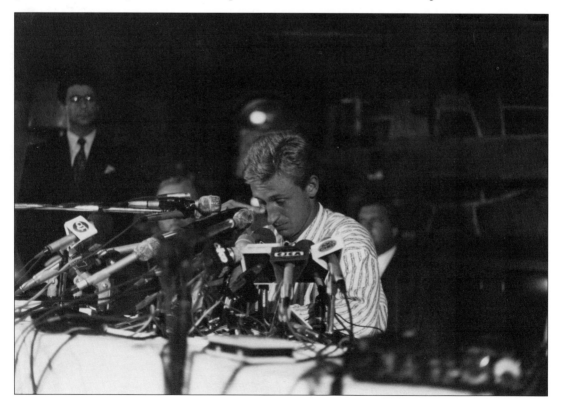

chasing Gretzky for the scoring title. "It's certainly going to be better for me."

Sure enough, Lemieux—the newly appointed captain of the Penguins—got off to a fast start in the 1988–89 season, registering a league-leading 41 points in his first 14 games. Coffey was firing on all cylinders, and heading toward his fourth 100-point-plus season. And in November, goalie Tom Barrasso, a former rookie of the year (1984) who was once voted the league's top netminder (1984), was acquired from Buffalo.

The Penguins challenged for the division lead. In October and again on New Year's Eve, Lemieux scored eight points in one game, a feat accomplished only 11 times before in league history; furthermore, Lemieux was only the second player ever to do it twice, after Gretzky. That New Year's Eve game, at home against the New Jersey Devils, also featured something that has to this day happened only this one time in an NHL game. Lemieux scored five goals, each one in a different man power situation: one goal came at even strength, another on a *power play,* an additional one while shorthanded, yet another off a penalty shot, and the final one into an empty net. Lemieux had scored for the cycle.

Lemieux also had nine *hat tricks* over the course of the season, and his 13 shorthanded goals were a new league record. He was in on 57 percent of his team's goals, a modern NHL standard. In the end he totaled 85 goals and 114 assists for 199 points, enough to easily beat out Gretzky for league scoring honors. His 85-goal season was the third best in NHL history (Gretzky had gotten 92 in 1982 and 87 in 1984), and his 199 points was the fifth most ever (Gretzky registered the top four).

The Penguins finished in second place, seven games over .500—their second best season ever. To make everything sweeter still, the Penguins were in the playoffs for the first time in Lemieux's five-year pro career. They opened with a four-of-seven series against the New York

Rangers, and disposed of them in four straight, outscoring them 19–11 in the process. The Penguins had won their first playoff series since 1979, and their first best-of-seven playoff series since 1970.

Next came the Philadelphia Flyers, who had finished the season well below Pittsburgh in the standings. The series proved difficult, and was tied at two games apiece going back to Pittsburgh for Game 5. Lemieux, though suffering from a stiff neck, exploded for a record-tying five goals. With three assists added on for good measure, Lemieux totaled eight points on that night, tying an NHL record established by New Jersey player Patrik Sundstrom just three nights before. The final score was 10–7, illustrating how Pittsburgh needed every single one of Lemieux's points to win the game. Yet paradoxically, Lemieux was totally shut down in Game 6, won by Philadelphia 6–2. That left the deciding Game 7, played before a wildly enthusiastic crowd at the Igloo. Lemieux scored to tie the game at 1–1, but neither he nor his teammates could do much else. They fell, 4–1, and lost the series, sending their fans home disappointed. Lemieux was disappointed, too, but said, "I know I'll drink from that Cup one day. I just know it."

In retrospect, it had been a great year for Lemieux and the Penguins. But not everything had come up roses. The team's new general manager, Tony Esposito, a former top goaltender from Sault Sainte Marie, Ontario, was in the habit of referring to the French Canadians as "frogs," and had even used the term in front of Lemieux. Writes Lawrence Martin:

> Esposito was frequently overheard commenting conde-scendingly or insultingly on aspects of the French-Canadian character. He allegedly went so far as to refer to Mario and other Quebeckers as "frogs." . . . Since the matter involved the team's lead player, it became an explosive behind-the-scenes issue. Bob Perno had talked

with Mario about the common perception outside of Quebec that Francophones were flashy but lazy players who
wouldn't backcheck. They agreed that this prejudice
would make life more difficult for him. They agreed that,
as a general rule, it was more difficult for a French-
Canadian playing in the NHL than for an English-
Canadian. But Mario never expected to be called a "frog"
to his face by the manager of his team.

Lemieux wanted Esposito fired. Eventually, he would get
his wish.

At the end of the 1989 season, Lemieux looked forward
to receiving his second straight Hart Trophy, but instead it
went to Gretzky for improving the Kings in his first year
in Los Angeles. Lemieux was upset. "Nothing in this
league makes sense," he said, one of many remarks in his
career that, although honest, was not as gracious as some
might have hoped.

Lemieux started 1989–90 by signing a new five-year
contract for $2.4 million a year, worth slightly more than
Gretzky's and the highest in the game. (Over the next few
seasons, they would leapfrog each other in terms of earn-
ing power, and by 1994 Gretzky would have the richest
annual salary in all of sports—$8.3 million per year.)

The Penguins got off to a slow start, and coach Gene
Ubriaco was fired—the third Penguins coach dismissed in
the slightly more than five years of Lemieux's career—
along with general manager Esposito. Ubriaco publicly
blamed Lemieux and Coffey for his firing; he was, in part,
correct, for Lemieux had clearly indicated he had no con-
fidence in Ubriaco. Esposito, too, was dismissed in part
because he had offended Lemieux. At the end of October
Lemieux started a point-scoring streak that was still going
at the January all-star break.

The 1990 all-star game was held in Pittsburgh. Before
the home fans, Lemieux scored three goals on his first
three shots and a fourth later on. He won another truck as
all-star MVP. But at the end of January his back, buttocks,

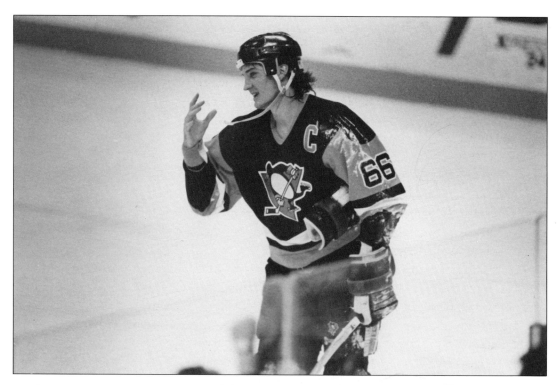

In 1990, the Penguins just missed qualifying for the playoffs. Lemieux had missed several regular-season games because of a herniated disk, and when he had it operated on in July he discovered he had developed an infection that would take months to heal. Lemieux thought his hockey days were over.

and legs began to ache, causing him tremendous pain. He played through the pain and continued to tally often, going for Gretzky's record of scoring a goal or an assist in 51 consecutive games, but eventually he had to wear a back brace.

Finally in mid-February Lemieux's point streak came to an end at 46 consecutive games when he could not finish a game in New York against the Rangers. As he sat out the next few games trying to recover from the excruciating back pain, Lemieux was hearing more criticism from the media. In a selfish effort to obtain an individual record, said his critics, he had hurt the team by continuing to play rather than resting. Now he was diagnosed with a herniated disk and would miss the stretch run of the regular season.

And while Lemieux was out the Penguins slumped. By the last game of the season they were on the brink of missing the playoffs; they needed at the very least a tie with Buffalo to qualify for postseason play. Lemieux came back for this vital game and scored a goal and an assist, but the contest still went into overtime. If the Penguins could only hold fast through the extra five minutes, they would be in the playoffs. But on an innocent play the puck went to a big Sabres defenseman named Uwe Krupp, who slapped it nonchalantly toward the Pittsburgh net from 90 feet away. The puck bounced on the ice unevenly, skipping past Barrasso and into the goal. Buffalo had won, and the Penguins missed the playoffs. Lemieux had scored 123 points in only 59 games, good enough for fourth in the league and easily the best points-per-game ratio, but the season was a dismal failure nonetheless.

With back pain continuing to plague Lemieux, he decided to have surgery. On July 11, 1990, the herniated part of the disk between the fourth and fifth lumbar vertebrae was removed along with some bone. It took him most of the summer to recover from the July operation, and just as soon as he felt he had recovered, the pain came back stronger than ever. Now the doctors told him he had developed an infection near the disk that had been operated on, and that the infection could cause his spine to deteriorate.

The Penguins' team physician, Charles Burke, told reporters that although the infection would likely respond to antibiotics, Lemieux's condition could nevertheless be termed "career-threatening." It would take at least three months, said Burke, for Lemieux to recover. Lemieux laid low during the recovery period. Reporters and fans wondered how he was taking this most serious crisis of his career so far. But neither Lemieux nor the Penguins would comment on his condition or on how he felt. Only Lemieux's closest friends knew that he was extremely worried, depressed, and afraid that his hockey career—the only thing he had really concentrated on for his entire life—might be over.

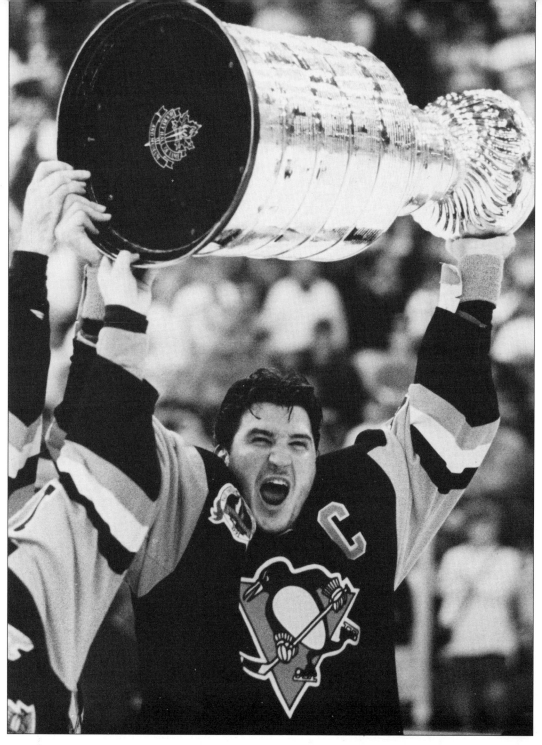

A jubilant Lemieux raises the Stanley Cup over his head after the Penguins defeated the Minnesota North Stars to win the 1991 championship, a first for the team.

7

DRINKING
FROM THE CUP

MARIO LEMIEUX did not talk to reporters for the nearly three months he was recovering from his back problems. After that time, he announced himself fit and thankful to be back. "I had some doubts that I would ever play again," he said.

Finally, after nearly a year's layoff, Lemieux returned to the ice on January 26, 1991, for a 6–5 victory in Quebec, scoring three assists. Nothing seemed to phase Lemieux. He played through what was left of the 1990–91 season with typical aplomb. His scoring was slightly down—an average of under two points a game—but scoring throughout the league was down from the high levels it had reached during the 1980s. He finished the regular season with 19 goals and 26 assists in just 26 games—a remarkable total considering what he had just been through. More incredible, perhaps, was that the Penguins won their first-ever division title that year. True, they finished the season with a modest eight games over .500, but they did so with Lemieux absent for two-thirds of the campaign.

The difference was the new front office installed after the firing of Esposito and Ubriaco. Craig Patrick—a former player and coach from the three generations of the Patrick family that at various times since 1926 had led the Rangers franchise—was the new general manager. At the start of 1990–91, he hired Scotty Bowman as head of player personnel—the coach with the most wins in NHL history and five-time victor of the Stanley Cup with the Canadiens in the 1970s. Patrick also hired "Badger" Bob Johnson, the 59-year-old longtime coach of the University of Wisconsin hockey team to be the new Penguins' coach. Wheeling and dealing, Patrick obtained several fine players: winger Joey Mullen from the Hell's Kitchen neighborhood of New York, the highest-scoring American in NHL history; centerman Ron Francis, former captain of the Hartford Whalers; tough Swedish defenseman Ulf Samuelsson; high-scoring defenseman Larry Murphy; and Bryan Trottier, captain and chief playmaker of the New York Islanders during their four-year run as Stanley Cup champions.

The Penguins were no longer a one-man team, dependent on Lemieux alone. That depth came in handy in the first round of the playoff series against New Jersey, when the Devils and the Penguins were tied at three games apiece going into the decider at the Civic Arena. Lemieux suffered a recurrence of his back pains, and, unable to bend over much less skate, was forced to retreat to the sidelines. Nevertheless, his teammates came through for a 4–2 victory, and the Penguins advanced. Lemieux was back for the next round, a five-game triumph over the Washington Capitals in which the most memorable feature was three straight winning goals from rugged winger Kevin Stevens. It was the first time ever that the Penguins had won two consecutive playoff series.

Their next hurdle was the Boston Bruins, who kicked off the semifinal series by winning the first two games at home. The key moment took place in Game 3, when Samuelsson checked Boston's high-scoring wingman, Cam Neely, severely injuring him. Although no penalty was called on the play, most observers believed that Samuelsson's knee smashing against Neely's thigh and felling him instantly was a dirty hit. It would take Neely well over a year to come back from the injury, from which he never fully recovered.

Whether or not the hit was the actual turning point in the Boston series is unclear, but it is true that the Penguins went on to win that game and the next three as well. With Lemieux setting up his teammates for goals time and time again, the Penguins had become one of the few teams in NHL history to rebound from a two games to zero deficit to win a series.

Lemieux scores a first-period goal against the Minnesota North Stars goalie Jon Casey in Game 1 of the 1991 Stanley Cup finals.

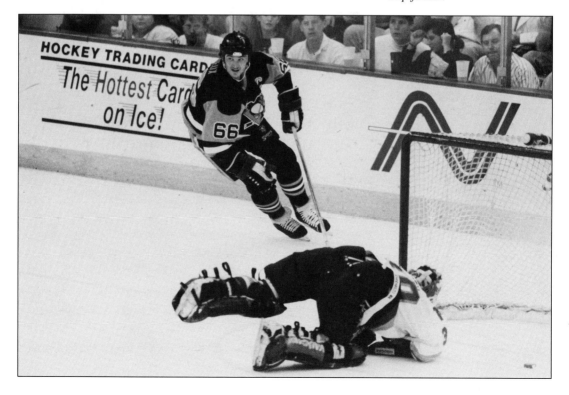

Now they were in the Stanley Cup final. Their opponents were the Minnesota North Stars, a team that had finished the regular season 12 games below .500 but had gotten hot in the playoffs. The Penguins, who had lost the first game in each of the prior three series, lost the first game of the final as well by a 5–4 score. But in Game 2 the Penguins bounced back. Leading 2–1 midway through the game, Lemieux split the North Stars defense pair, then deked the goalie out of position before depositing the puck in the net. Pittsburgh went on to win 4–1.

Lemieux's back spasms returned before Game 3, forcing him to miss the contest. The Penguins duly lost. At his hotel, Lemieux was given a stiff new bed for more back support, and at the rink, a trainer was assigned the task of tying his skate laces so he would not have to bend over. The precautions worked, and Lemieux scored early in Game 4 to help Pittsburgh achieve a series-tying 5–3 victory. Back at the Igloo for Game 5, Lemieux scored a goal and set up two others, all in the first period, to pace the Penguins to a 6–4 win and pull within one game of lifting the Stanley Cup. Game 6 at Minnesota was a blowout—an 8–0 triumphal procession for the Penguins.

The Pittsburgh Penguins had finally won the Stanley Cup. According to hockey tradition, the two teams lined up at center ice and shook hands. Then the Stanley Cup was carried out to center ice and presented to Pittsburgh's captain, Lemieux. Beaming, he held it aloft, and, with the Minnesota crowd applauding politely, the team started a victory lap around the rink, passing the three-feet-high, 36-pound silver trophy among themselves so that each player held it. Into the dressing room they went to congratulate one another, sip champagne from the Cup's silver bowl, and embrace their wives and girlfriends, who had been invited in for the special occasion (indeed, it was unusual to see so many women in the locker room of a championship team, whose postgame celebrations are usually all-male affairs). Among the women in the room were

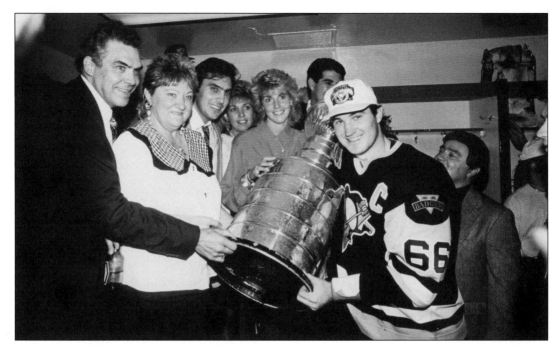

Nathalie Asselin and Pierrette Lemieux, who shared Mario's joy during these special moments.

"You dream of this," said Lemieux. "But it's even better in real life than it is in your dreams."

Many hockey critics and fans had said that Lemieux could not be considered a winning player unless he had won a Stanley Cup. Lemieux maintained that he did not care what people said about him as long as he had the respect of his teammates.

Fellow Penguin Paul Coffey said, "The criticism has to have hurt him a little. But I know it would hurt him more if he had thought his teammates believed any of that stuff. He was going to hear it until he won a Stanley Cup. It was unfair, but that's the way it goes."

Johnson told reporters, "Dominating a Stanley Cup victory was the one thing left for Mario to achieve in establishing himself as one of the truly great players in the history of hockey. If there were any questions left, I think he has supplied the answers."

Lemieux poses with the Stanley Cup in the locker room after the Penguins' 1991 victory. Celebrating with Lemieux are his parents, Jean-Guy and Pierrette (left), and his girlfriend, Nathalie Asselin (center).

Lemieux had finished with 44 points in 23 playoff games, the second highest single-year playoff point total of all time; the highest was—who else's?—Gretzky's 1985 mark of 47 points in 18 games.

As icing on the cake, Lemieux received the Conn Smythe Trophy as playoff MVP. Three days later, a huge celebration for the Stanley Cup champions was held at Pittsburgh's Point State Park. More than 40,000 people came to see the Penguins and the Cup. Bryan Trottier, his enthusiasm as bright as ever despite this being the fifth time he had won the game's ultimate prize, looked out over the cheering crowd and boomed, "Enjoy it, Pittsburgh. Enjoy it, baby."

Afterward, Lemieux took the Cup back to Ville Emard, set it on the kitchen table of the family house on rue Jorgue, and greeted a long line of well-wishers. Later, as is the practice with this most famous of North America's sports trophies, the Cup was engraved with the names of all the Penguins players.

That summer, it was time for the fifth renewal of the quadrennial Canada Cup tournament. Lemieux chose to sit out the competition because of his tender back, and this time, few begrudged him his decision.

Pittsburgh's coach, the sunny, upbeat Johnson, whose personal motto, "It's a great day for hockey," had become a Pittsburgh catchphrase, would go to the tournament as coach of the U.S. team. Returning to Pittsburgh following the Americans' last tune-up game before the contest in late August 1991, Johnson fell ill with what was believed to be a stroke. But tests revealed that he had cancer— specifically, several brain tumors. The outlook was grim. "I saw him about a week and a half ago," said Lemieux. "He was the same old Badger everybody knows. It's scary, really sad."

Yet despite his condition, Johnson scribbled out a start- ing lineup and tactical notes for the United States's open- ing game in the tournament. A few days later Lemieux offered more on what Johnson meant to him: "What he's done for this city and this hockey club in one year is pretty incredible. Nobody thought we'd win the Cup, but with Bob Johnson, anything was possible."

Johnson underwent brain surgery, which made the left side of his body paralyzed. He was unable to speak, but his mind was still alert. When he learned that the Devils had signed a top blueliner, he wrote a note to Patrick that read, "Uh-oh, New Jersey's got a great defense." Eventually he was flown back to his home in Colorado Springs. Strapped to a medical gurney, he even attended a Penguins exhibition game in Denver and greeted the players. After the start of the season, the Penguins ceremoniously raised the Stanley Cup banners at the Igloo, and Johnson sent along a statement: "I walked in the arena one year ago and noticed that there were no championship banners here. Well, tonight it is great to have these championship banners raised for the fans of Pittsburgh, signifying that we have reached the top of the mountain."

On November 26, 1991, Johnson died. "Bob was a great teacher," remembered Lemieux. "And more than anything else, he taught us how to win."

With Bowman filling in as interim coach—he pointedly never took Johnson's title—the Penguins started the 1991–92 season slowly once again. Early in the year, Lemieux suffered a bad cut above his eye when New Jersey defenseman Viacheslav Fetisov got careless with his stick, an offense for which Fetisov was suspended for five games. Halfway through the campaign, Lemieux's chronic back pain returned, and again he was forced to think of what his life after hockey might be like.

"If it's going to hurt me for the rest of my life," he said of his aching back, "it's not worth it. I think everybody is frustrated because we can't figure out what's causing the pain."

Burke commented that the unpredictable nature of the ailment left Lemieux depressed: "It becomes so mentally difficult because just when he thinks things are going to get better, the pain comes back."

Teammate Ron Francis said, "You don't want to live 30 years of your life in pain. We'd rather see Mario enjoy life than go through the aggravation he is now."

Lemieux was relieved when doctors diagnosed the ailment as a herniated muscle, which was far less serious than another disk or spinal problem. More rest improved his condition, but because he never knew how he would feel when he woke up the next morning, he was frustrated, and

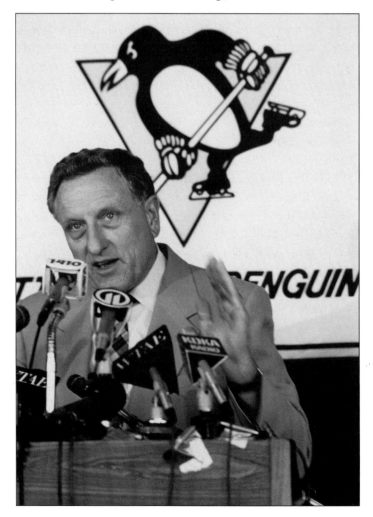

Beloved Pittsburgh coach "Badger" Bob Johnson, whose motto was, "It's a great day for hockey," died of brain cancer on November 26, 1991.

this showed on the ice. Playing on January 26, 1992, he was outraged by what he saw as goon tactics in a game against Washington. Lemieux complained that the NHL was a "garage league" for allowing such methods to go unpunished. He said, "There are so many rules that are stupid in this league." The NHL fined him $1,000 for this remark.

In mid-February, after another enforced layoff due to back woes, Lemieux went on a scoring tear. On March 14, he scored his 400th career goal. On March 22, he recorded his 1,000th career point, making him the second fastest player, after Gretzky, to reach that milestone. On March 26, he added his 600th career assist. In 1992, he also shot past Gretzky and teammate Kevin Stevens and finished first in scoring with 44 goals, 87 assists, and 131 points in only 64 games, winning his third Art Ross Trophy.

"He's the best player in the world," said Francis of Lemieux. "And people who refuse to recognize him as such are missing the boat."

Still, the Penguins had not had such a good regular season, finishing just seven games over .500. Did they have what it takes to be Cup champions again? One thing they did not have for the opener of their series against Washington was Lemieux, who was out with a shoulder injury. Pittsburgh lost 3–1, then lost again 6–2 with Lemieux back in action. In Game 3 at the Igloo, he put on a one-man show with three assists followed by three goals in a 6–4 win, but then the Penguins dropped Game 4. Facing elimination, they rallied to win Game 5, then Lemieux turned his magic on again with two goals and three assists in a come-from-behind 6–4 Game 6 victory. In the decider, Lemieux scored the go-ahead goal, a short hander, and helped the Penguins to victory from the brink of extinction.

"I give all the credit to Mario Lemieux," said Washington's Al Iafrate of Lemieux, who scored 17 points in six games. "Period. Exclamation point."

Next came the Rangers. With Pittsburgh up one game to zero and leading Game 2 1–0, the Penguins went on a first-period power play. Lemieux had the puck along the *boards* when New York's Adam Graves, trying to whack Lemieux in the hands to make him lose the puck, took a two-handed slash at the Penguin captain's gloves.

Lemieux immediately crumpled to the ice. The Madison Square Garden fans booed, assuming that Lemieux was faking an injury. But he was indeed hurt, with a broken metacarpal bone in his left hand. Graves received only a two-minute penalty on the play, and the Rangers went on to win the game. Graves, however, was subsequently suspended for four games due to his actions. Lemieux, it was believed, was gone for the duration of the playoffs.

The Penguins soldiered on regardless, losing Game 3 in overtime and trailing 4–2 in the third period of Game 4. But then a lucky break came their way. Francis shot a long, routine *slap shot* from the blue line that Rangers goalie Mike Richter missed, drawing the Penguins within one goal. They came back to tie and won the game in overtime, then were victorious the next two games as well to take the series, all without Lemieux.

Pittsburgh next faced Boston, and incredibly, Lemieux returned for Game 2 of the series. And despite his still-broken hand, he scored two goals and an assist. The Penguins went on to crush the Bruins in four straight games. They were in the Cup final for the second straight year. Their opponents were the Chicago Black Hawks, one of whose defensemen, Steve Smith, noted that Lemieux "will tear us apart if we allow him to run loose." That comment proved prophetic.

The Black Hawks jumped out to a 4–1 lead in Game 1, but with five minutes left on the clock, they clung to a one-goal edge. At that point the Penguins' big young Czech, Jaromir Jagr—whose size, reach, and looks make him resemble Lemieux so closely that fans are fond of pointing out that the name "Jaromir" is an anagram for

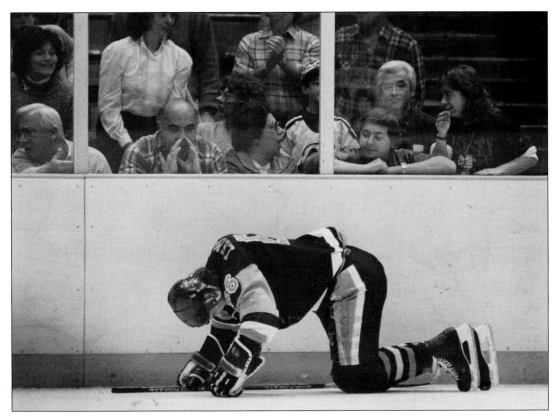

"Mario Jr."—scored one of the most fabulous goals in hockey history. Bringing the puck into the Chicago end, he stood along the left-wing boards, offered the puck to one Black Hawk, took it away, shifted past another player and then another, and shot it past the netminder for the tying goal.

More heroics followed, as a Black Hawk was penalized for pulling Lemieux down with only 18 seconds to go in regulation time, giving Pittsburgh a power play. Murphy took a shot off the *face-off* that the Black Hawk goalie kicked out, but Lemieux was there to bury the rebound with 13 seconds left. Pittsburgh won. "We never quit," Lemieux said afterward.

Chicago coach Mike Keenan, who had praised Lemieux so extravagantly after the 1987 Canada Cup,

In Game 2 of the 1992 playoffs against the New York Rangers, a player slashed at Lemieux's gloves, breaking a metacarpal bone in his left hand. The fans at Madison Square Garden booed Lemieux, believing he was faking an injury.

Penguins captain Mario Lemieux leads his teammates on the ice as he carries the Stanley Cup. It is a long-standing tradition for the captain of the winning team to be the first to skate around the rink holding the Cup. The Penguins won their second straight NHL championship in 1992 against the Chicago Black Hawks.

accused Lemieux of diving in front of the Black Hawk player to draw the late penalty. He called Lemieux "an embarrassment to himself, to the game, and to the players he's playing with."

Lemieux replied on the ice in Game 2 by scoring the go-ahead and insurance goal in a 3–1 victory. The series moved to Chicago for Game 3, which was won by the Penguins, 1–0. Lemieux scored a goal and two assists in a 6–5 Game 4 victory that closed out the series in four straight games. For the second year in a row, the Penguins had won the Stanley Cup. And for the second straight year, Lemieux won the Conn Smythe Trophy as playoff MVP.

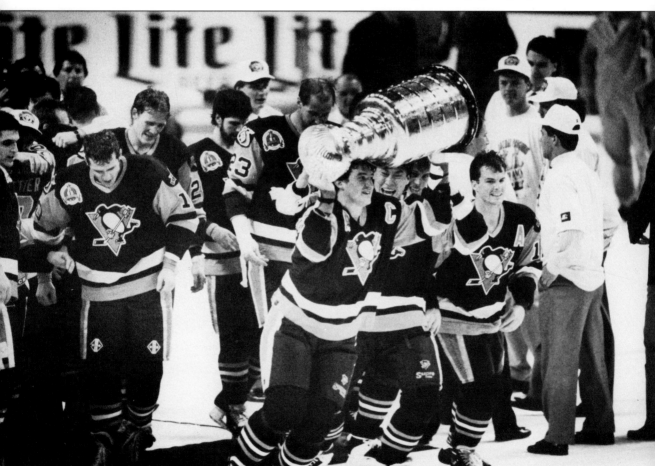

Keenan even indirectly retracted his earlier remark about Lemieux. "We were just beaten by a better club," he said. "They have youth, experience, and the greatest player in the world."

A few days later, some 40,000 Pittsburghers gathered in the city's Three Rivers Stadium for the Stanley Cup celebration. A persistent rain failed to dampen the proceedings, and Lemieux watched and laughed along with the crowd as Trottier grabbed the Cup and slid around the slippery tarpaulin like a schoolboy.

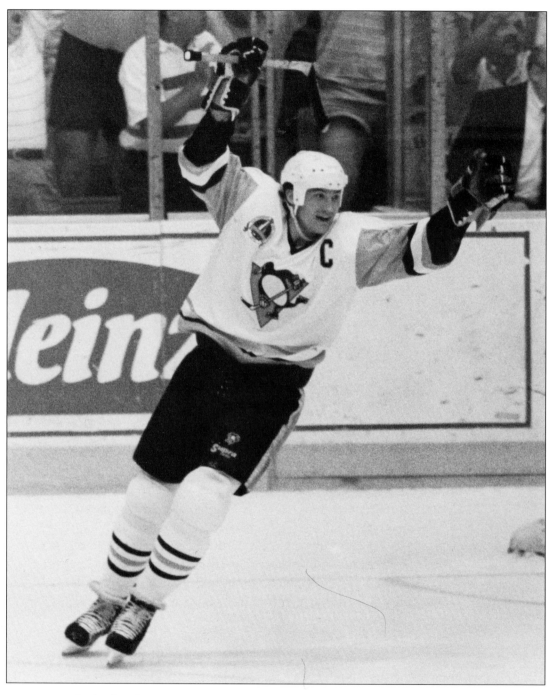

By leading his team to two Stanley Cup championships, Lemieux engraved his name in the annals of hockey history, assuring his place as one of the greatest hockey players of all time.

8

SUPER MARIO

BACK PAIN GONE, his name engraved on the Stanley Cup twice in a row, and with a new seven-year contract worth $6 million a year, Lemieux started the 1992–93 campaign on top of the world. And now it looked like he might supplant Gretzky both literally and figuratively. Gretzky was out of play with a career-threatening disk problem of his own, and Lemieux was on a scoring jag that might break the Great One's all-time mark. With 46 points in 16 games, Super Mario—another one of his nicknames—was on pace to smash Gretzky's single-season record of 215 points.

In November, though, Lemieux was involved in an alleged rape case. He and former teammate Dan Quinn got together after a game in Minnesota and went back to their hotel with two women they had met at a bar. The players and their female companions adjourned to Lemieux's room, where, one of the women alleged, Quinn raped her.

Quinn asserted that the sex was consensual. In the end no charges were brought against Quinn, but many took a dim view of Lemieux's part in the affair, particularly because Asselin was home in Pittsburgh, pregnant.

The fallout from the case quickly faded into the background, however, when Lemieux held the early January 1993 press conference to announce he had a nodular lymphocytic form of Hodgkin's disease. Now all other matters, like Lemieux's quest for Gretzky's record being stalled at 104 points in 40 games, were secondary.

"I'll be back when I'm 100 percent cured," Lemieux told the assembled reporters, who remembered only too well coach Bob Johnson's losing battle with brain cancer, and the winning battle Tom Barrasso's two-year-old daughter, Ashley, fought with neuroblastoma, another form of cancer.

Lemieux's radiation treatments began on February 1, after his unrelated lung infection cleared up. For the treatment, Lemieux lay beneath a face mask and a lead shield that covered much of his body to protect vital organs from the massive doses of radiation he received. To align the shield in the correct place each day, small dots were tattooed on Lemieux's chest. Lying in a high-energy linear accelerator, he then received two or three minute-long blasts of radiation, 50 times more powerful than a normal X ray. The blasts were aimed at his neck. This routine was repeated five times a day for five weeks.

"When I had the mask on," said Lemieux, "I thought, 'This is why I'm here, because of the cancer.' That's when I really thought about it. But as soon as I got out of there and got into my car, I let it go."

The usual side effects of such treatment are sore throat, damage to salivary glands that causes "cotton mouth," and, most commonly, fatigue. Karl Nelson, a New York Giants football player who received radiation treatment for Hodgkin's in 1987, told author Robert Brody that the sessions severely drained him. "As an athlete, you're used

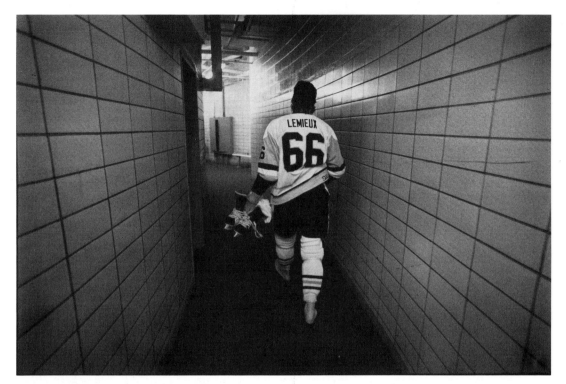

to pushing yourself through tough situations," Nelson said. "I knew I would be able to tolerate radiation because I was in good shape, and I was used to functioning when I was tired."

The same applied for Lemieux, who knew that Nelson succeeded in coming back to the Giants for a brief time before ultimately having to retire. Lemieux also knew about U.S. Olympic wrestler Jeff Blatnick, who was treated for Hodgkin's in 1982 and bounced back from radiation and surgery to win a gold medal at the 1984 Olympics. Blatnick tried again in 1988, but the cancer recurred. The second round of treatments, however, cured him.

Lemieux lost his sense of taste during the treatments, but did not experience as much fatigue as he had expected. Just two weeks after the treatments began, he was skating with the Penguins at practices. On March 2, he received

Lemieux walks down the corridor to the locker room during a game. When he was diagnosed with Hodgkin's disease, Lemieux thought he would never again be able to play hockey.

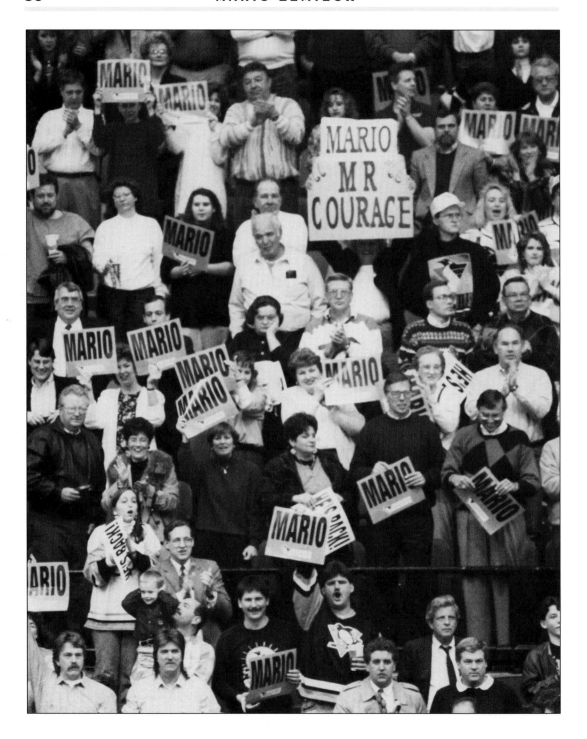

his final radiation blast, which was so strong it burned his neck. Lemieux got right up from the table, joined a friend who drove him to the airport, and caught a plane to Philadelphia.

That night at the Philadelphia Spectrum, the Penguins were playing the Flyers. And when Mario Lemieux stepped on the ice in his black and gold uniform, the Flyer fans greeted him with a 90-second standing ovation. Incredibly, he scored a goal and an assist during the game. A few nights later he played his first home game, and the Civic Arena crowd paid him a moving tribute. Fans held up hundreds of preprinted signs reading "Mario"; "He's Back!"; and "Mario, Mr. Courage."

Lemieux went on a scoring binge in the weeks that followed, pulling off such feats as back-to-back four-goal games, a five-goal game, and a 16-game scoring streak in which he tallied 51 points. Still a bit wobbly from the radiation treatments, Lemieux offered the explanation, "Sometimes the more tired I feel, the better I play."

Pat LaFontaine, his tormentor from QMJHL days and now a Buffalo Sabre, had taken over the scoring lead in Lemieux's Hodgkin's-enforced absence, but now Lemieux was bearing down on him. Lemieux caught up with his rival with less than a month left in the regular season, and wound up with his fourth scoring title on 69 goals, 91 assists, and 160 points in only 60 games; he also finished with a league-high rating of plus 55, illustrating how rarely opponents scored when he was on the ice. All in all, Lemieux had accomplished one of the most— perhaps *the* most—amazing individual performances in hockey history.

Biographer Lawrence Martin wrote:

His teammates spoke of how they drew strength from his performance. . . . They watched him in his phenomenal late-season surge, knowing that he was handicapped, not at his peak, but still doing it better than anyone else. They knew that if the fates would only let him, Mario could take

OPPOSITE:
When Lemieux returned to the ice after undergoing radiation therapy for Hodgkin's disease, hockey fans were thrilled to see him skating again. At his first game back, the Flyers' fans in Philadelphia gave him a 90-second standing ovation. At home a few nights later, the Penguins' fans raised signs hailing the return of their idol.

the sport to levels higher than anyone else ever had—as high as only he could imagine.

The Penguins had won 11, lost 11, and tied 2 with Lemieux out of action. When he was in the lineup, the club had 45 wins, 10 losses, and 2 ties. It was the Penguins' best regular-season performance ever, and for garnering the most points of any team during the NHL's regular schedule, they added the President's Trophy to their two Stanley Cup triumphs.

In search of their third straight Cup, the Penguins opened the playoffs against the New Jersey Devils. Lemieux led the way once more, racking up five goals and four assists as the Penguins coasted in five games—the ninth straight series the once-flightless birds had won. In the next series, the Penguins faced the plucky Islanders.

Lemieux missed most of Game 1, all of Game 2, and parts of games 3 and 4 because of back spasms before returning pain-free to lead the Penguins to a Game 5 win. Pittsburgh was up 3 games to 2 against the underdog team from Long Island, New York, but Lemieux was again hobbled in Game 6 and the Penguins lost. He tried traction treatments for Game 7 but they did not help. The Penguins rallied to tie the match in the final minutes, but could only watch in horror as the Islanders won in overtime. The Penguins' Cup run was over.

Meanwhile, Gretzky, recovered from his own serious back problems, was leading the Kings to the Stanley Cup final. But this time Number 99 did not overshadow his younger rival. Lemieux capped his eventful hockey year by collecting his second Hart Trophy as the league's most valuable player, his third Lester B. Pearson Award as players' MVP, and the Masterton Trophy for perseverance and dedication to the game. Lemieux thus became the first player ever to win the Hart, Smythe, Ross (scoring champion), and Masterton awards.

The 1992–93 season was a time of drama for Lemieux, with periods of anguish and pain interspersed with plea-

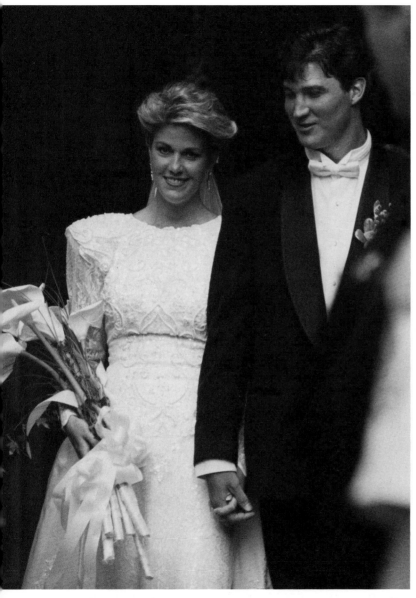

Lemieux married his longtime sweetheart, Nathalie Asselin, on June 26, 1993, in Montreal. Two months earlier Asselin gave birth to their daughter, Lauren.

sures and blessings. Late in 1992, immediately before he was diagnosed with cancer, he and his fiancée, Nathalie, had purchased a new home in Sewickley, a small, quiet town 12 miles west of Pittsburgh. On April 29, 1993, Lemieux's daughter, Lauren Rachel, was born. And on

June 26, he and Asselin were married in a ceremony in Montreal attended by friends and family. In July, he announced the formation of the Mario Lemieux Foundation, to support cancer research programs to organizations and hospitals in the United States and Canada. In late July, he was back in the hospital to repair another herniated muscle in his back—just the usual routine for Mario Lemieux.

The 1993–94 campaign was not a particularly successful one for Lemieux or the Penguins. Able to play in only 22 games because of back pains, he scored 32 points and, of course, did not challenge for the scoring title, which went to the rejuvenated Gretzky. The Penguins dropped off a bit to only the third-best record in the league, then lost their opening-round playoff series to the Capitals.

Through it all Lemieux felt out of step and fatigued. After losing the final game to the Capitals, he told reporters he was considering retirement. He would decide, he said, over the summer.

It was later revealed that Lemieux was suffering from anemia, a condition in which the blood is deficient in red blood cells, the cells that carry oxygen to the tissues. This condition expresses itself in chronic fatigue. The anemia had apparently arisen as a result of the radiation treatments for Hodgkin's that Lemieux had undergone in early 1993, and also, perhaps, as a result of a dozen cortisone injections he had received for back pain in 1991. Anemia, a much more serious problem when someone with Hodgkin's disease develops it than when a healthy person does, left Lemieux with little leg strength to play hockey.

In the off-season Lemieux played in various charity golf tournaments amid rumors that he would sit out the following campaign, or perhaps retire from hockey altogether before reaching age 29. The rumors gained force in July when the Penguins acquired French Canadian scoring star

Luc Robitaille from the Los Angeles Kings in exchange for Rick Tocchet and a second-round draft choice. A few days later they added help at Lemieux's position, center, by picking up John Cullen, who had been a big scorer with Pittsburgh a few years before. Then they re-signed star forwards Jaromir Jagr and Tomas Sandstrom.

Meanwhile, Lemieux was tested for Hodgkin's, and no recurrence was found. Furthermore, his anemic condition had subsided. But still the fatigue remained.

Finally, on August 29, 1994, Lemieux announced at a Pittsburgh press conference that he would not retire— at least not yet. Instead, he would sit out the 1994–95 season to recover from the fatigue that had been plaguing him for so long.

"I need to regain the strength I had two years ago," said Lemieux. "I can't train the way I want. I get tired very quickly. The stamina is not the same as it was at the end of last season.

"It's been very difficult the last couple of years, but I want everybody to know I still love the game of hockey," continued Lemieux. "It's not a hockey issue. It's a health issue."

"Over the past four years," Lemieux's agent, Tom Reich, said, "he's had major back surgery, acute osteomyelitis [the bone infection that affected his verte-brae], Hodgkin's, and additional back surgery. During those four years, he has found the time to win two scoring titles, an MVP, two Stanley Cup MVPs, two division titles—with a lot of help from his friends."

As for whether he would come back after the season, Lemieux was uncertain. "I don't want to come back until I can play the way Mario Lemieux can play," he said, referring to himself in the third person. "If I feel I'm not able to go on the ice and be close to 100 percent, another decision will have to be made." He added that if he was able to play 60 games a year, he would "try and come back.

*Mario Lemieux proudly
stands behind the trophies
he collected for the 1992–93
NHL season: the Ross Trophy
(center) as the NHL's scoring
leader; the Hart Trophy
(right) as the NHL's most
valuable player; and the
Masterton Trophy (left) for
perseverance, sportsmanship,
and dedication to hockey.*

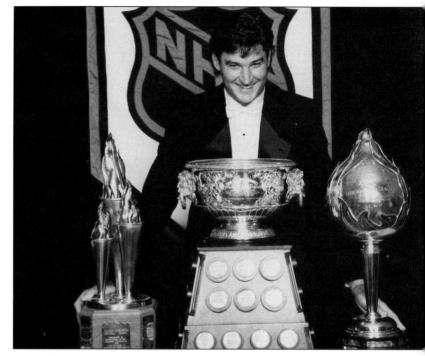

I'm going to miss going to the rink every day," said Lemieux. "I'm going to miss being around the guys."

Asked whether Lemieux was still battling Hodgkin's, Reich was adamantly optimistic. "Mario's prognosis for Hodgkin's is excellent," said Reich. "He will never have another bout with that again."

Neil Smith, general manager of the New York Rangers, who just two months before had won their first Stanley Cup in 54 years, summed up the feelings of the entire sports world. "He is simply one of the all-time greats, and I've seen Gordie Howe, Bobby Orr, Bobby Hull, and Jean Béliveau," Smith told *USA Today*. "If he retires, no one can ever doubt Lemieux. He has won two Stanley Cups, plus all of his personal accomplishments."

And indeed, the chances seemed better than remote that within a few more months Lemieux would decide to hang up the skates for good. "Right now," he said, "my health is a lot more important than hockey."

That was certainly true, and all the more so for having been said by Mario Lemieux, who had played through cancer and everything else like he has played through defenses all his life. Fans in Pittsburgh and beyond can count themselves fortunate to have been able to see the big Montrealer with the loping stride cruising down the ice, baffling defenders with sudden shifts of weight from side to side, fooling goaltenders with the long reach of his stick. And they will never forget the joy he brought when he raised his hands in that characteristically nonchalant way as the red goal light flashed and the bright easy grin spread across his face. Perhaps they would see more of that still.

"Lemieux." Translate it into English and you will discover what it means: "The best."

GLOSSARY

back-check	to skate back toward one's own goal while defending against the opposing team's offensive players
blueliner	another word for a defenseman; the two blue lines on the floor of the ice break the playing surface into three sections to indicate the neutral zone and each team's end zone
boards	the wood surface, topped with glass, that surrounds the playing area
bodycheck	to legally hit an opponent with a shoulder or hip to slow or stop him
breakaway	a player skating quickly toward the goalie in an attempt to score
center	the middleman of the three players who make up the offensive line
defensemen	the two players (right and left) whose main job is to help the goalie prevent opponents from scoring
deke	a fake by the person carrying the puck to maneuver around an opposing player
drop pass	a move in which the player in control of the puck suddenly leaves the puck where it is so that a teammate following closely behind can scoop it up
face-off	the dropping of the puck between the sticks of two opposing players to start or resume play; there are eight spots and a center circle where the game can be restarted
forward	a player who attacks in the offensive zone; includes the right wing, left wing, and center
hat trick	three goals scored by a player in one game
linesman	the official who restarts the game with a face-off after determining which rules have been broken; there are three officials for each game—one referee and two linesmen who assist him
neutral zone	center ice, between the two blue lines

penalty	a punishment for violating the rules that involves suspension from the game for a specified period of time; in rare cases, a misconduct penalty may be given to a player, resulting in possible ejection from the game
periods	the three 20-minute segments of play that make up a hockey game
playmaker	a player, usually a center, who is able to set up plays and give signals that lead to a goal
power play	a play during which one team has a penalty and, as a result, the opposing team has more players on the ice; the team with the advantage sends players to the opposition's goal to try to score
slap shot	a shot to the net accomplished by bringing the stick back, raising it to shoulder height, and then quickly pushing the puck ahead; usually a player's fastest shot
wingmen	the men in the forward line, one playing on the right side of the ice and the other playing on the left side

APPENDIX

AMATEUR AND PROFESSIONAL RECORD

Season Team	League	Regular Season					Playoffs				
		Gms.	G	A	Pts.	Pen.	Gms.	G	A	Pts.	Pen.
81-82–Laval . . . . .QMJHL		64	30	66	96	22	18	5	9	14	31
82-83–Laval . . . . .QMJHL		66	84	100	184	76	12	14	18	32	18
83-84–Laval . . . . .QMJHL		70	133	149	282	92	14	29	23	52	29
84-85–Pittsburgh . . . . .NHL		73	43	57	100	54	–	–	–	–	–
85-86–Pittsburgh . . . . .NHL		79	48	93	141	43	–	–	–	–	–
86-87–Pittsburgh . . . . .NHL		63	54	53	107	57	–	–	–	–	–
87-88–Pittsburgh . . . . .NHL		77	70	98	168	92	–	–	–	–	–
88-89–Pittsburgh . . . . .NHL		76	85	114	199	100	11	12	7	19	16
89-90–Pittsburgh . . . . .NHL		59	45	78	123	78	–	–	–	–	–
90-91–Pittsburgh . . . . .NHL		26	19	26	45	30	23	16	28	44	16
91-92–Pittsburgh . . . . .NHL		64	44	87	131	94	15	16	18	34	2
92-93–Pittsburgh . . . . .NHL		60	69	91	160	38	11	8	10	18	10
93-94–Pittsburgh . . . . .NHL		22	17	20	37	32	6	4	3	7	2
NHL totals		599	494	717	1211	618	66	56	66	122	46

HONORS AND AWARDS

Calder Memorial Trophy (rookie of the year): 1985

Hart Trophy (NHL's most valuable player): 1988, 1993

Bill Masterton Trophy (perseverance, sportsmanship, and dedication to hockey): 1993

NHL All-Rookie Team: 1985

NHL All-Star first team: 1988, 1989, 1993

NHL All-Star second team: 1986, 1987, 1992

Lester B. Pearson Award (most valuable player chosen by the NHL players): 1986, 1988, 1993

Art Ross Trophy (NHL's scoring leader): 1988, 1989, 1992, 1993

Conn Smythe Trophy (playoff most valuable player): 1991, 1992

FURTHER READING

Brody, Robert. *Edge Against Cancer: The Athlete's Advantage Against Cancer and How To Gain It.* Waco, Texas: WRS, 1993.

Diamond, Dan, ed. *The Official National Hockey League 75th Anniversary Commemorative Book.* Toronto: McClelland & Stewart, 1991.

———. *The Official National Hockey League Stanley Cup Centennial Book.* Buffalo, NY: Firefly Books, 1992.

Fischler, Stan, and Shirley Fischler. *Everybody's Hockey Book.* New York: Scribners, 1983.

Germain, Georges-Hebert. *Overtime: The Legend of Guy Lafleur.* New York: Viking, 1990.

Klein, Jeff Z., and Karl-Eric Reif. *The Klein and Reif Hockey Compendium.* Toronto: McClelland & Stewart, 1987.

Martin, Lawrence. *Mario.* Toronto: Lester, 1993.

Molinari, Dave. *Best in the Game: The Turbulent Story of the Pittsburgh Penguins' Rise to Stanley Cup Champions.* Champaign, Illinois: Seamore, 1993.

Morrison, Scott. *Fire on Ice: Hockey's Greatest Series.* Downsview, Ontario: Pulse Books, 1987.

National Hockey League. *Official Guide and Record Book.* Chicago: Triumph Books. Published annually.

Reilly, Rick. *Gretzky: An Autobiography.* Toronto: HarperCollins, 1990.

Romain, Joseph, and James Duplacey. *Hockey Superstars.* London, Ontario: WH Smith, 1991.

Sonmor, Jean. *Mario Lemieux: Hockey's Gentle Giant.* Toronto: Macmillan Canada, 1989.

CHRONOLOGY

1965   Mario Lemieux born in the village of Ville Emard, Montreal, Canada, on October 5

1968   Begins playing hockey at age three, showing incredible skill for a young child

1971–1980   Plays on various levels of the Ville Emard hockey team; wins several awards and leads his team to the championships each year

1981   Lemieux is picked first in the Quebec Major Junior Hockey League (QMJHL) draft to play for the Laval Voisins

1982   Chosen for the national team in the world junior championships in Leningrad, Soviet Union; named to QMJHL All-Star second team for the 1982–83 season

1983   Starts off season by scoring 35 points in his first seven games; named Canadian Major Junior player of the year and wins the Michael Brière, Jean Béliveau, Michael Bossy, and Guy Lafleur trophies

1984   At 18 years old, Lemieux is chosen as an underage junior by the Pittsburgh Penguins in the first round of the National Hockey League (NHL) entry draft; selected as NHL rookie of the year (Calder Memorial Trophy); named to NHL All-Rookie team

1985   Finishes the season with 43 goals and 57 assists to his credit, the third highest total for any rookie in NHL history; plays in the world championships at Prague, Czechoslovakia, assisting in a victory over the Soviet Union; named All-Star Game most valuable player

1986–87   Penguins start season with a seven-game winning streak; Lemieux is ranked second in scoring only to his friend and rival, Wayne Gretzky; plays for Team Canada in the Canada Cup Tournament against the Soviet Union, in which Gretzky sets Lemieux up for a sudden-death goal, clinching the victory for Canada

1988   Appointed captain of the Penguins, who win their first playoff series since 1979 and their first best-of-seven playoff series since 1970; wins the Hart Trophy as the NHL's most valuable player

1990   Lemieux has surgery in July to correct a herniated disk in his back; the surgery causes him to miss the first 50 games of the season, and leaves him uncertain about his future in hockey

1991   Returns to the ice on January 26, assisting in a victory for the
         Penguins; the Penguins make the Stanley Cup playoffs against
         the Boston Bruins, and then triumph over the Minnesota North Stars
         to take the Stanley Cup for the first time ever; Penguins coach Bob
         Johnson has surgery for brain cancer; Johnson dies on November 26

1992   Lemieux continues to suffer from back spasms, but assists the
         Penguins in winning their second Stanley Cup in a row against the
         Chicago Black Hawks; wins his third trophy as leading scorer in the
         NHL; in March records his 400th goal, 600th assist, and 1,000th point;
         signs a new seven-year, $6 million contract with the Penguins

1993   Holds a press conference on January 12 to announce he has Hodgkin's
         disease; Lemieux undergoes first radiation treatments from February
         through March, still managing to attend Penguin practices; returns
         to the lineup on March 2 and scores a goal and an assist; finishes the
         season with his fourth scoring title and an incredible league-high rating
         of plus-55; daughter, Lauren, born on April 29; marries longtime
         girlfriend Nathalie Asselin on June 26, in Montreal

1994   On August 29 announces that he will sit out 1994-95 season to recover
         from anemia, fatigue, and back problems

INDEX

PICTURE CREDITS

Jeff Z. Klein is sports editor at the *Village Voice* in New York City, and with Karl-Eric Reif he is co-author of *The Klein & Reif Hockey Compendium.* Mr. Klein resides in New York City.

Jerry Lewis is the National Chairman of the Muscular Dystrophy Association (MDA) and host of the MDA Labor Day Telethon. An internationally acclaimed comedian, Lewis began his entertainment career in New York and then performed in a comedy team with singer and actor Dean Martin from 1946 to 1956. Lewis has appeared in many films—including *The Delicate Delinquent, Rock a Bye Baby, The Bellboy, Cinderfella, The Nutty Professor, The Disorderly Orderly,* and *The King of Comedy*—and his comedy performances continue to delight audiences around the world.

John Callahan is a nationally syndicated cartoonist and the author of an illustrated autobiography, *Don't Worry, He Won't Get Far on Foot.* He has also produced three cartoon collections: *Do Not Disturb Any Further, Digesting the Child Within,* and *Do What He Says! He's Crazy!!!* He has recently been the subject of feature articles in the *New York Times Magazine,* the *Los Angeles Times Magazine,* and the Cleveland *Plain Dealer,* and has been profiled on "60 Minutes." Callahan resides in Portland, Oregon.